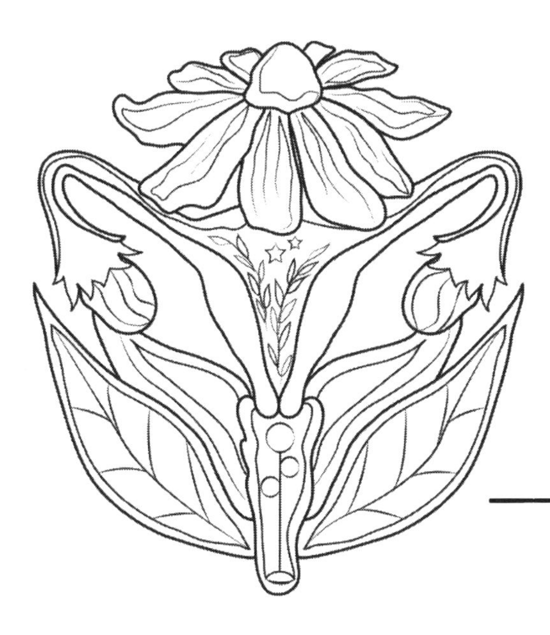

This Book Belongs to

____

Thank you for your purchase

To ensure that you have the best experience using this coloring book and to prevent bleeding, although the illustrations are on one-side, we highly recommend coloring using pencils.
If you are going to use any kind of ink that may cause bleeding through out the papers, we recommend tearing out the coloring pages or using a buffer page. (you can find blank buffer pages at the end of the book.)

I wish you a speedy recovery and wish you a life full of happiness...

Having a hysterectomy is probably an emotional rollercoaster, from worries about the surgery and worries about how life will be after to the relief and the blessing that the tumors and the pain were gone, plus hope that life will be much easier and less painful.

I'd like to share my mother's hysterectomy story with you: My mother was in her early 40s, and I was almost a teenager when tumors were discovered in her uterus.
I remember all the worries we went through.
I remember how she questioned her femininity and how her life would be like.
I remember how she feared aging so quickly.
I remember how it took her few weeks to fully recover from surgery.
I remember how she was blessed by having our family and friends around her.

I'm blessed by how she is so happy and healthy now, many many years after her surgery.
By going through these tough times, you are saving your life and trying to do your best to have a healthy and happy life.
Your main goal during your recovery is only YOU ...
Try to have the support systems you deserve, surround yourself with loving friends and caring family, and take care of yourself. Self-care, especially in those moments, is mandatory.
Self-care can be done in many ways, one of which is coloring.
Hope this coloring book will put a smile on your face and support you in your recovery.

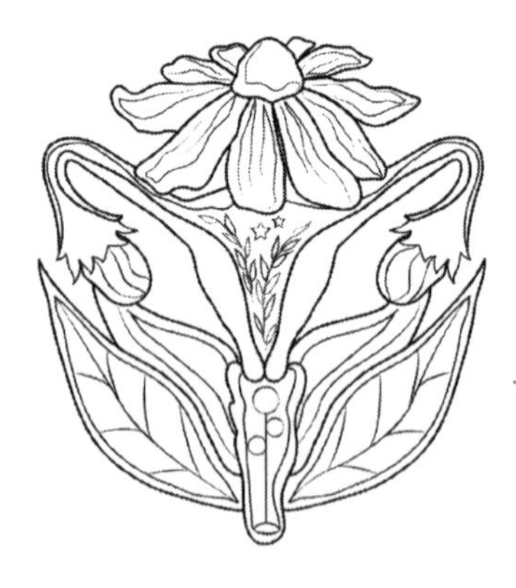

This page is intentionally left blank to avoid color bleeding.

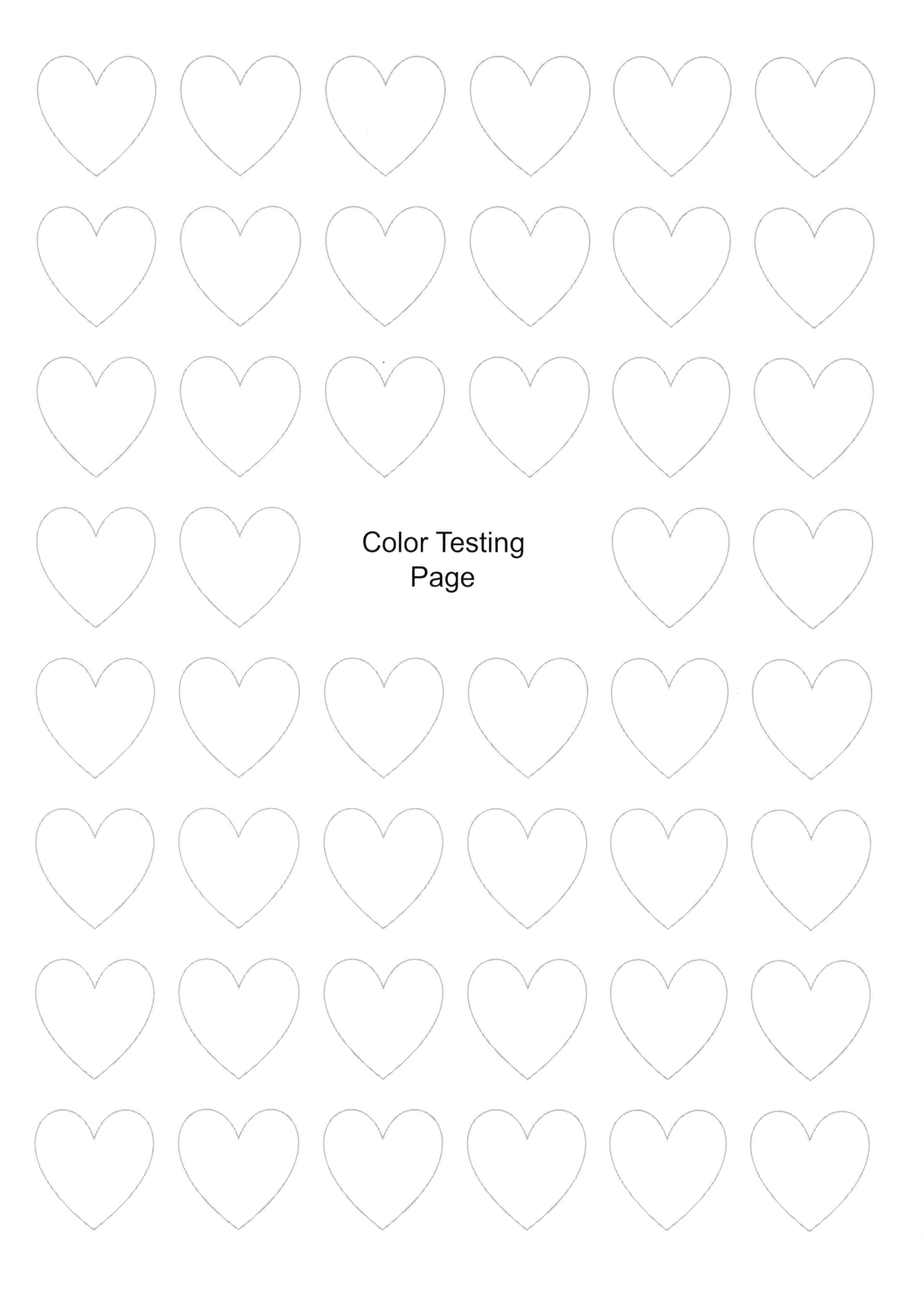
Color Testing
Page

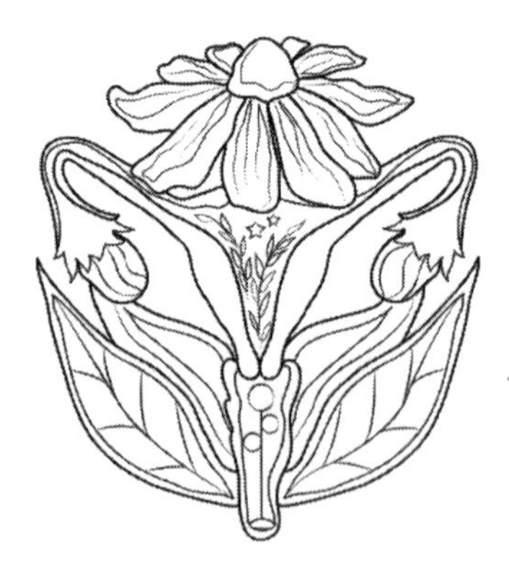

This page is intentionally left blank to avoid color bleeding.

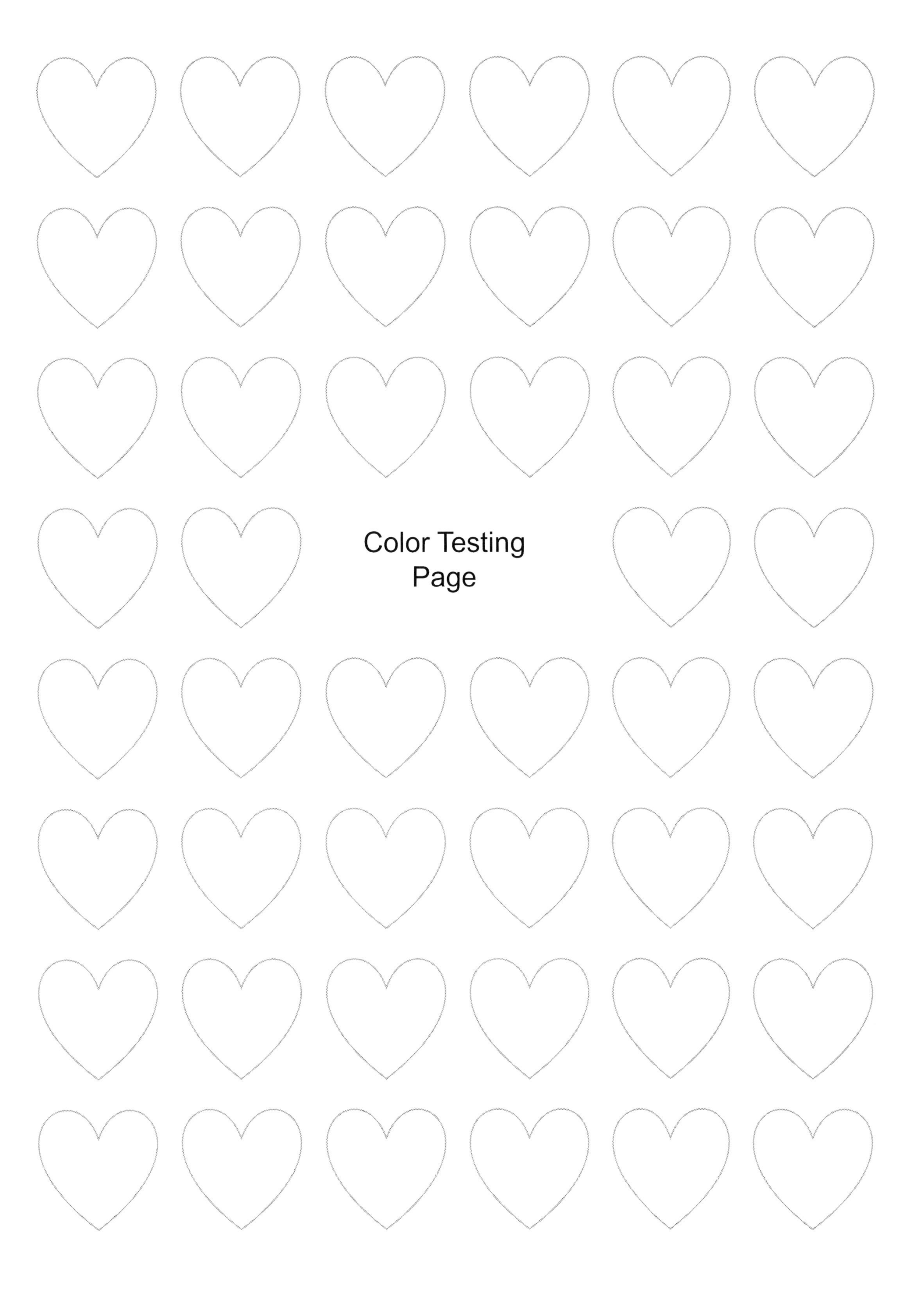
Color Testing
Page

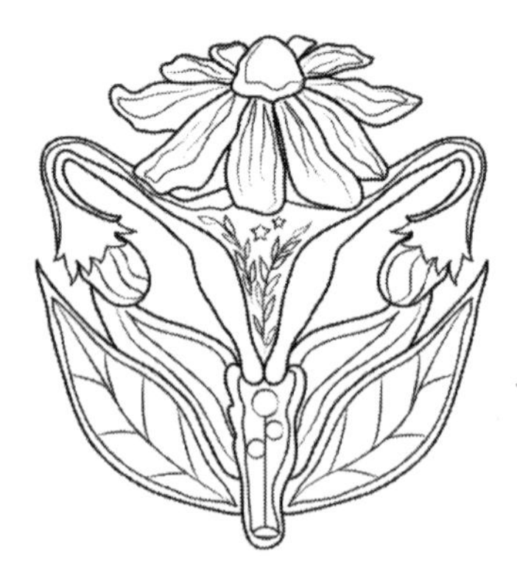

This page is intentionally left blank to avoid color bleeding.

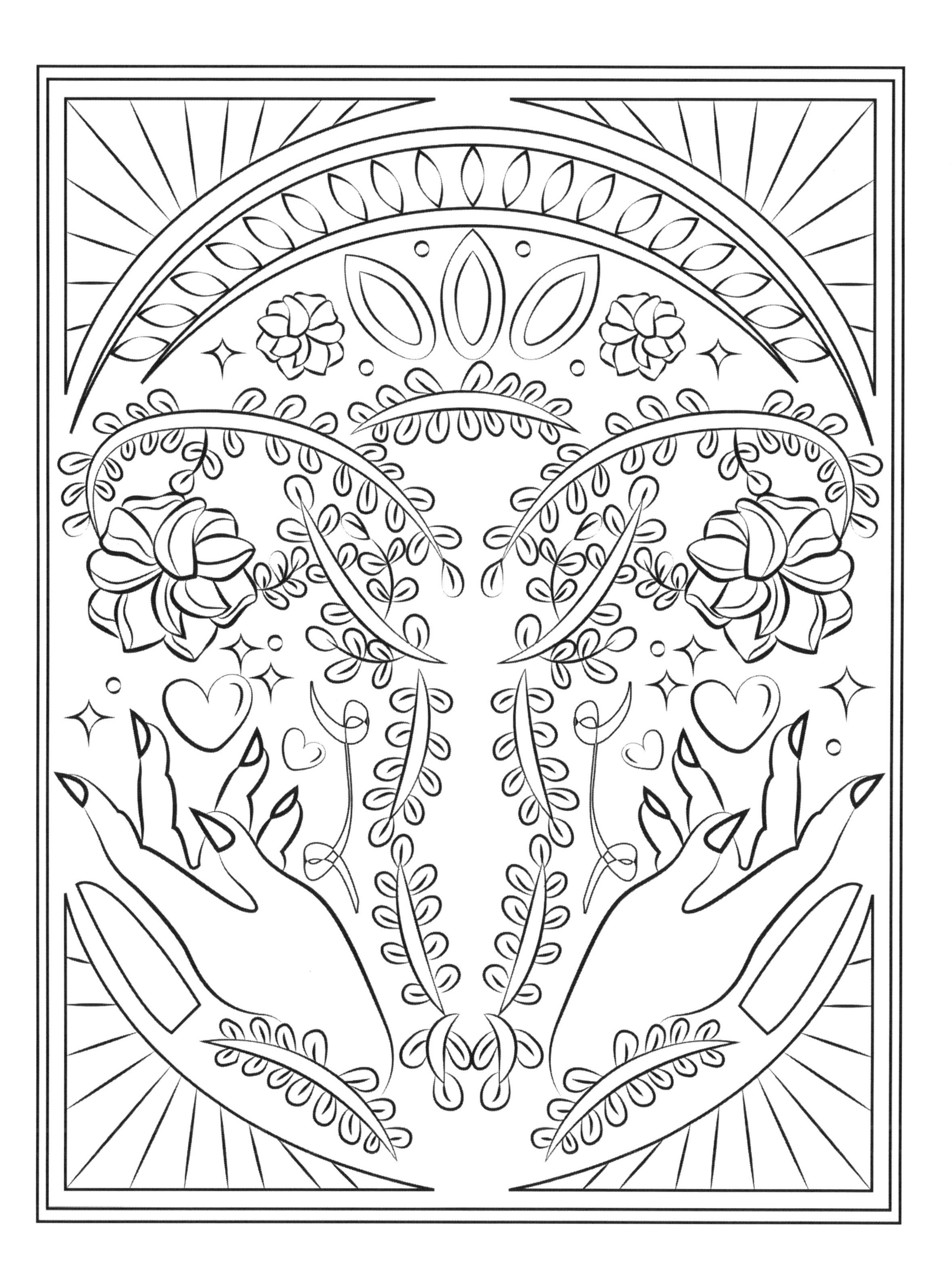

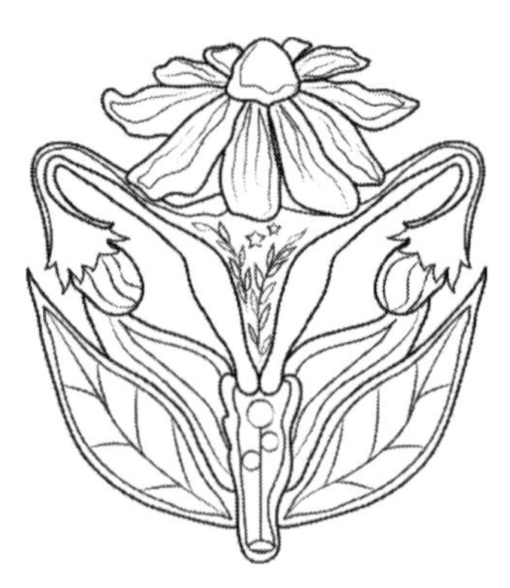

This page is intentionally left blank to avoid color bleeding.

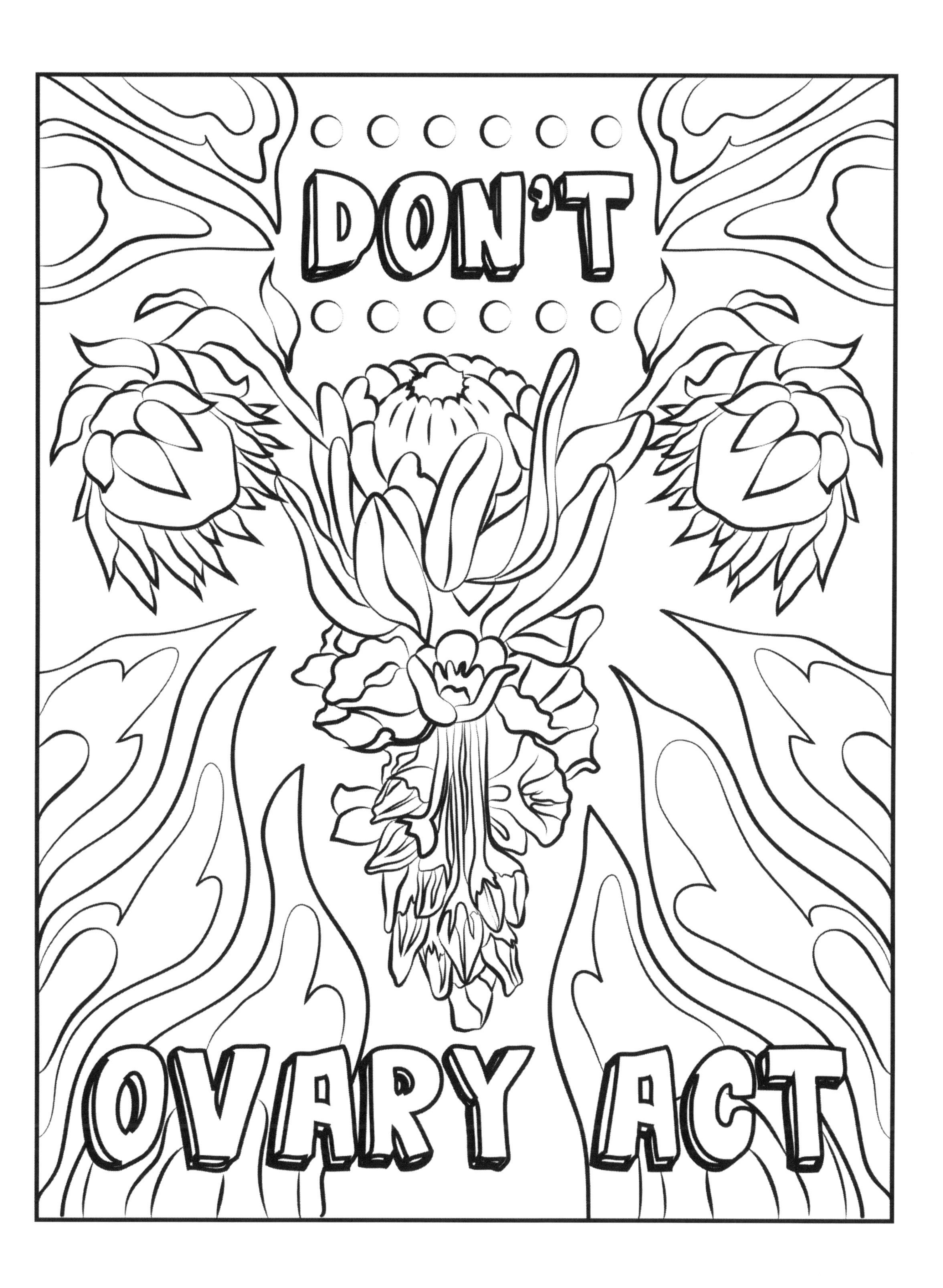
DON'T
OVARY ACT

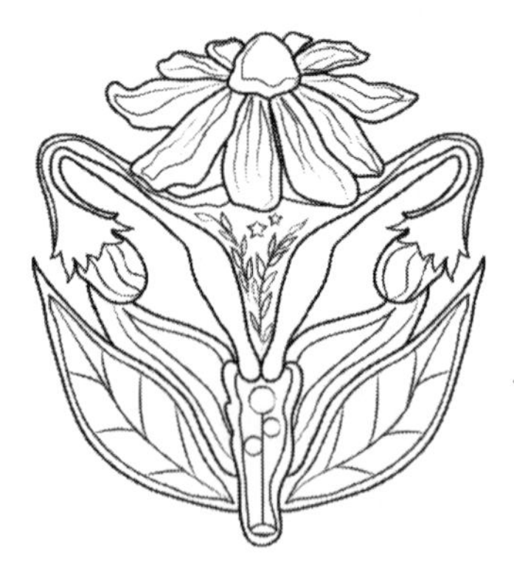

This page is intentionally left blank to avoid color bleeding.

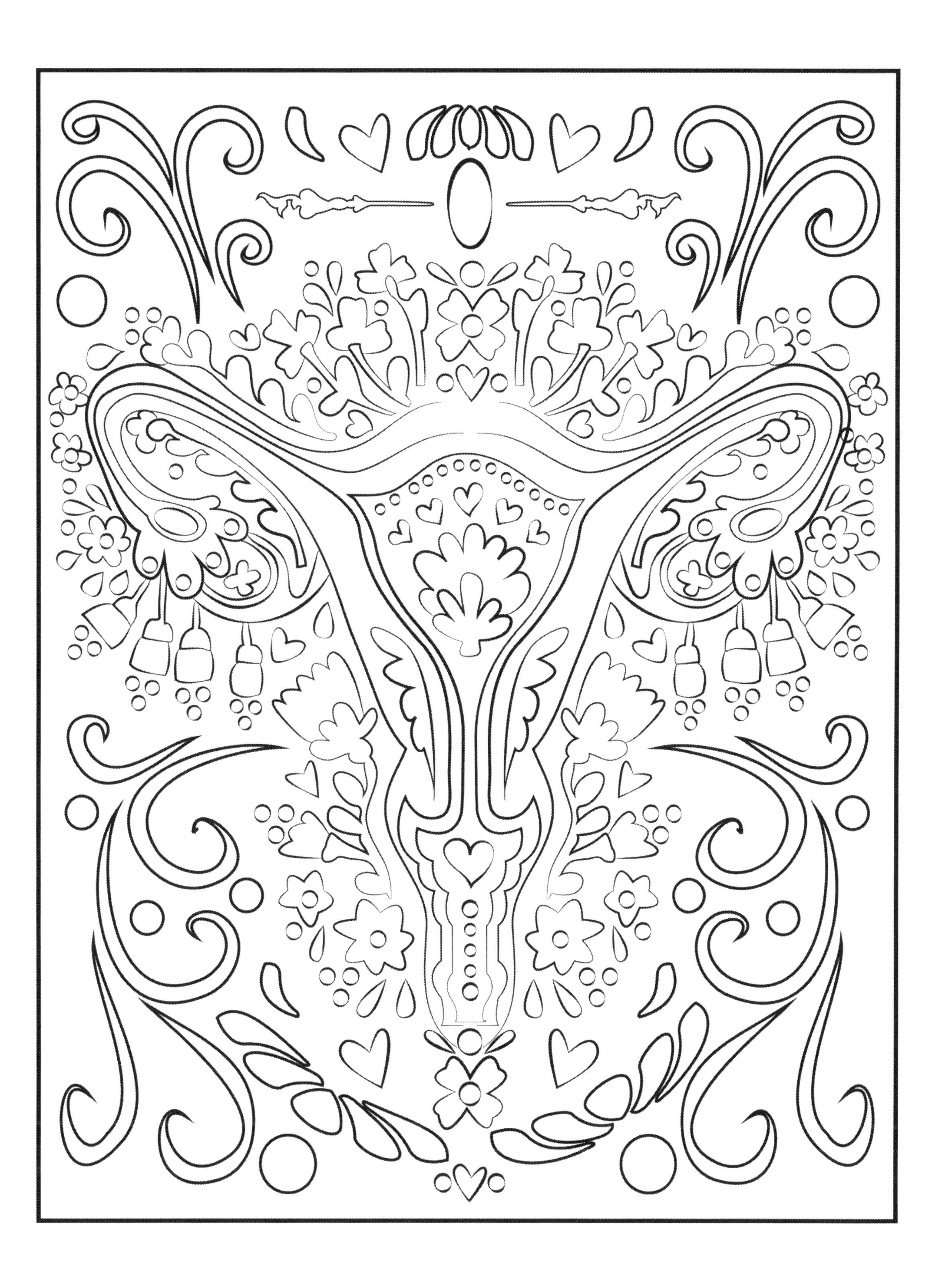

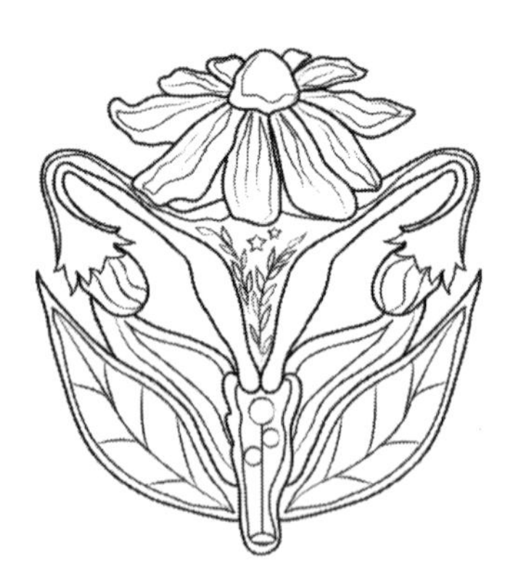

This page is intentionally left blank to avoid color bleeding.

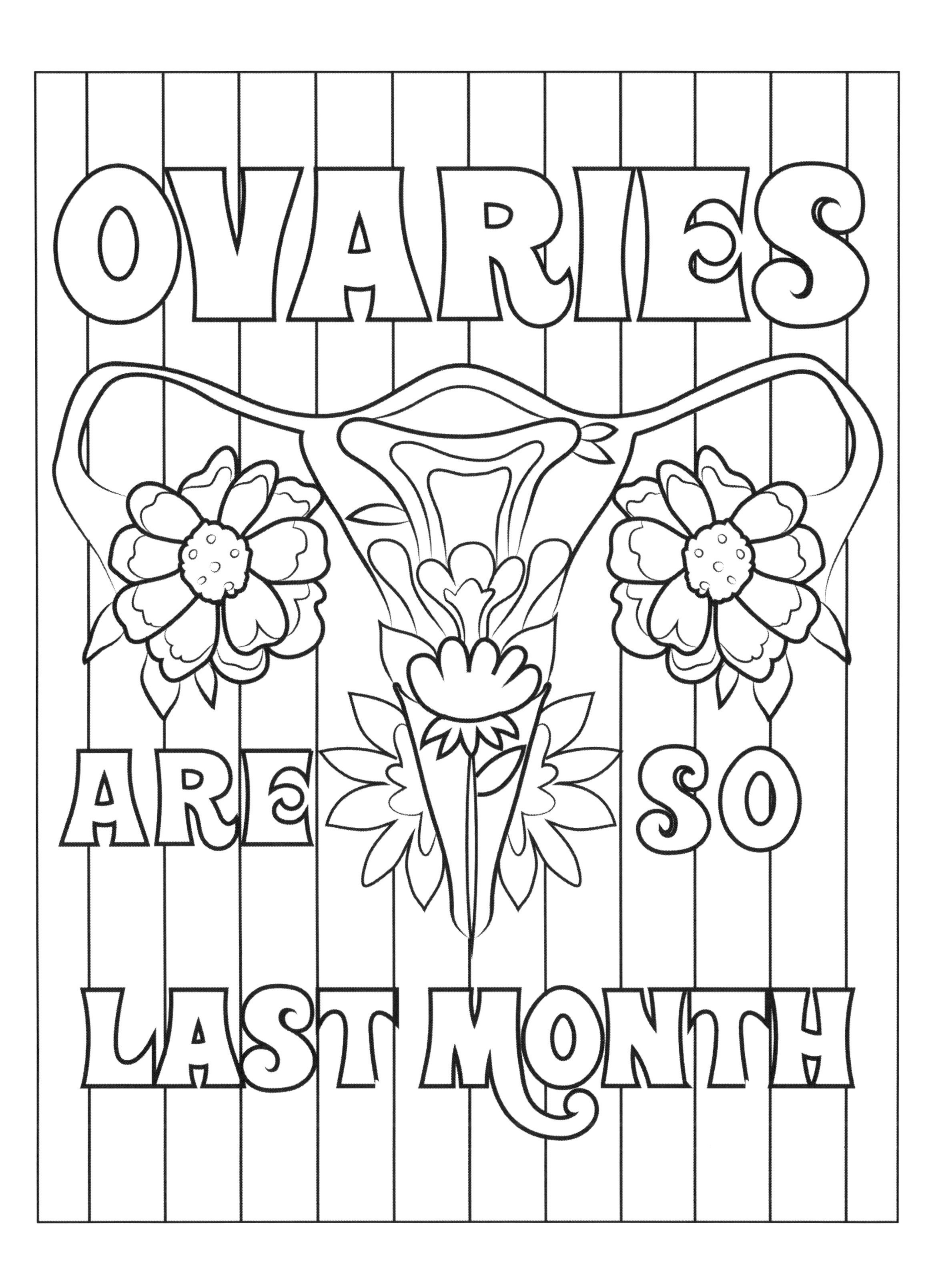
OVARIES
ARE SO
LAST MONTH

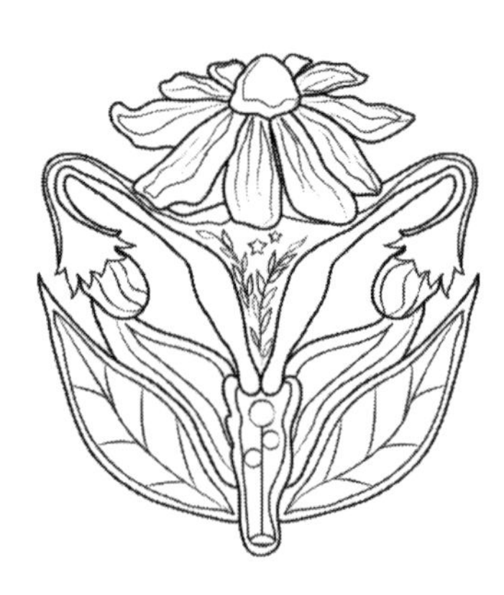

This page is intentionally left blank to avoid color bleeding.

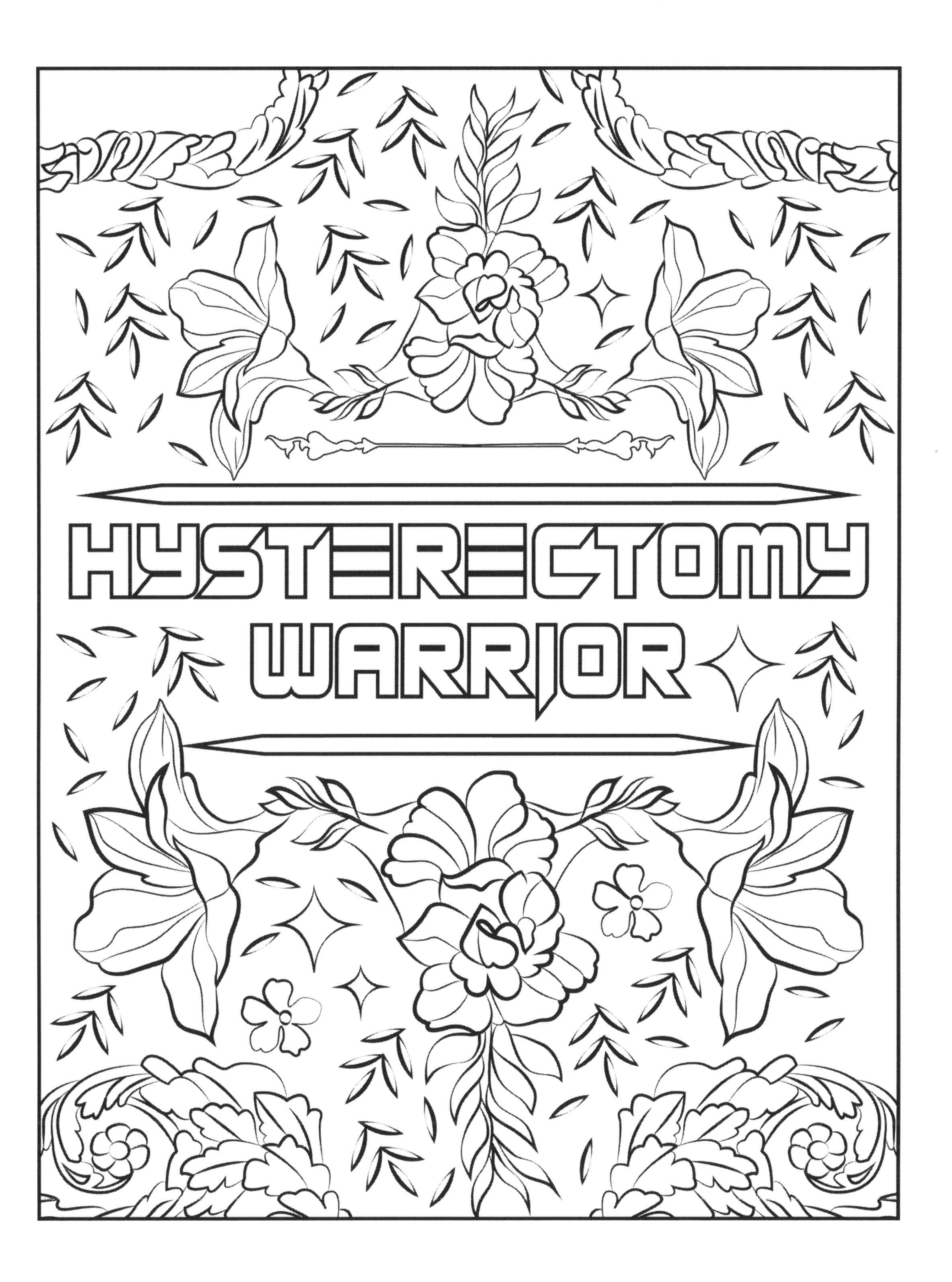
HYSTERECTOMY
WARRIOR

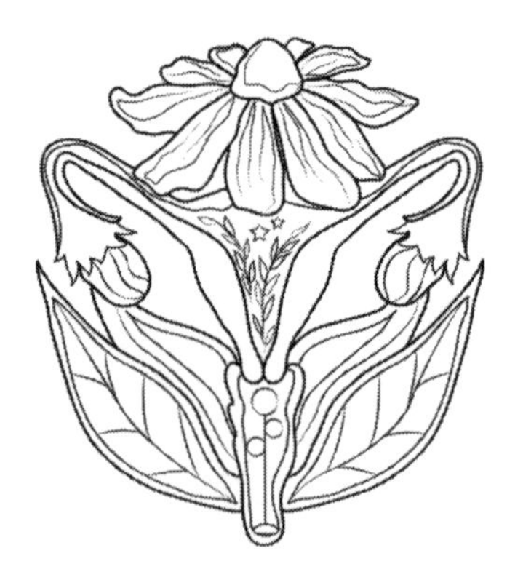

This page is intentionally left blank to avoid color bleeding.

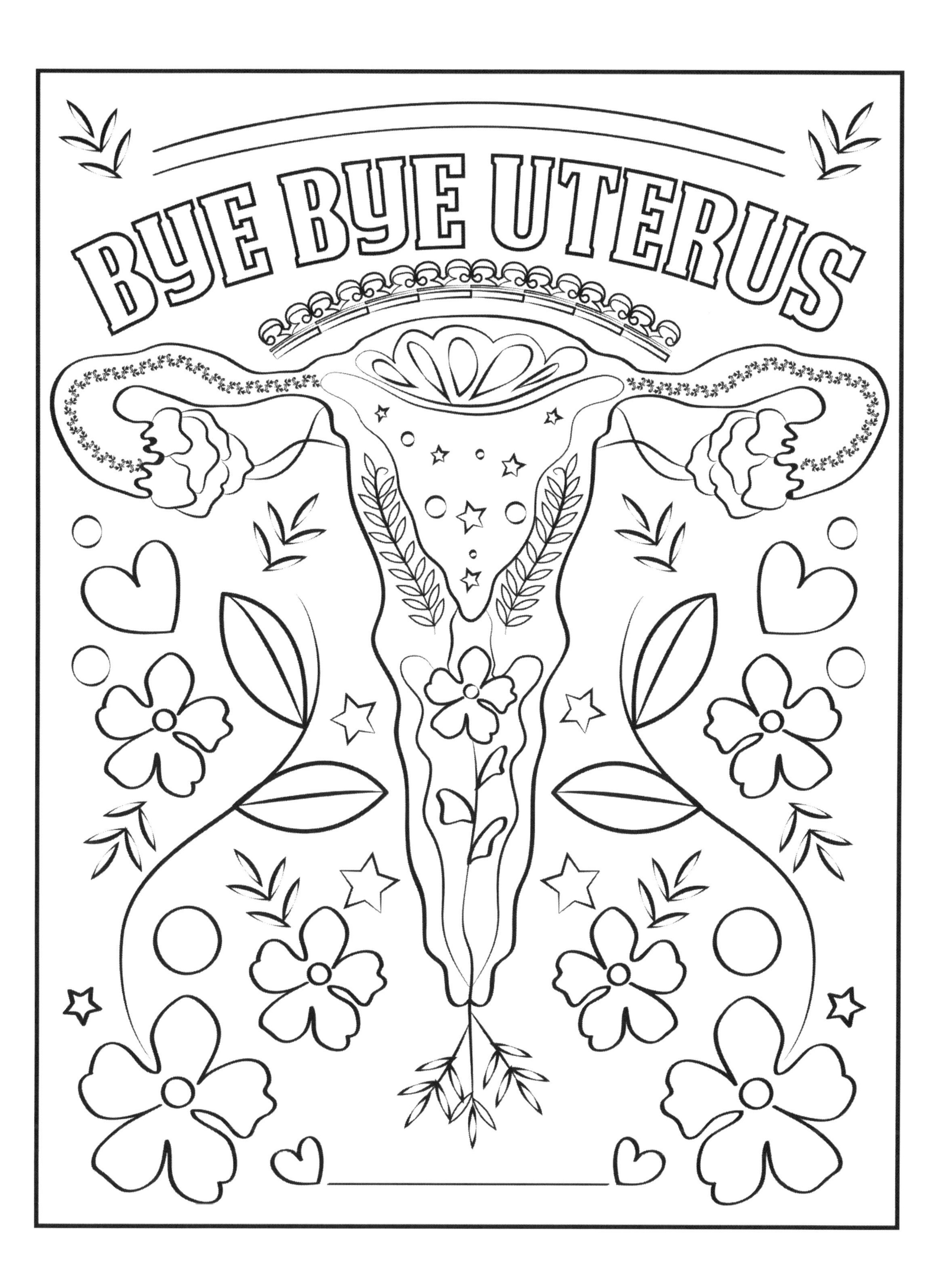
BYE BYE UTERUS

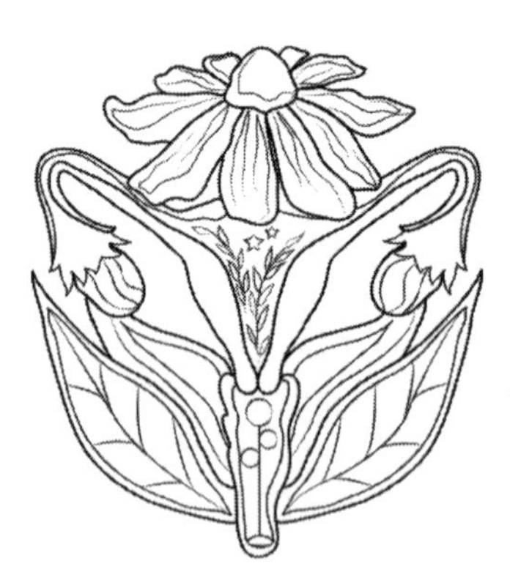

This page is intentionally left blank to avoid color bleeding.

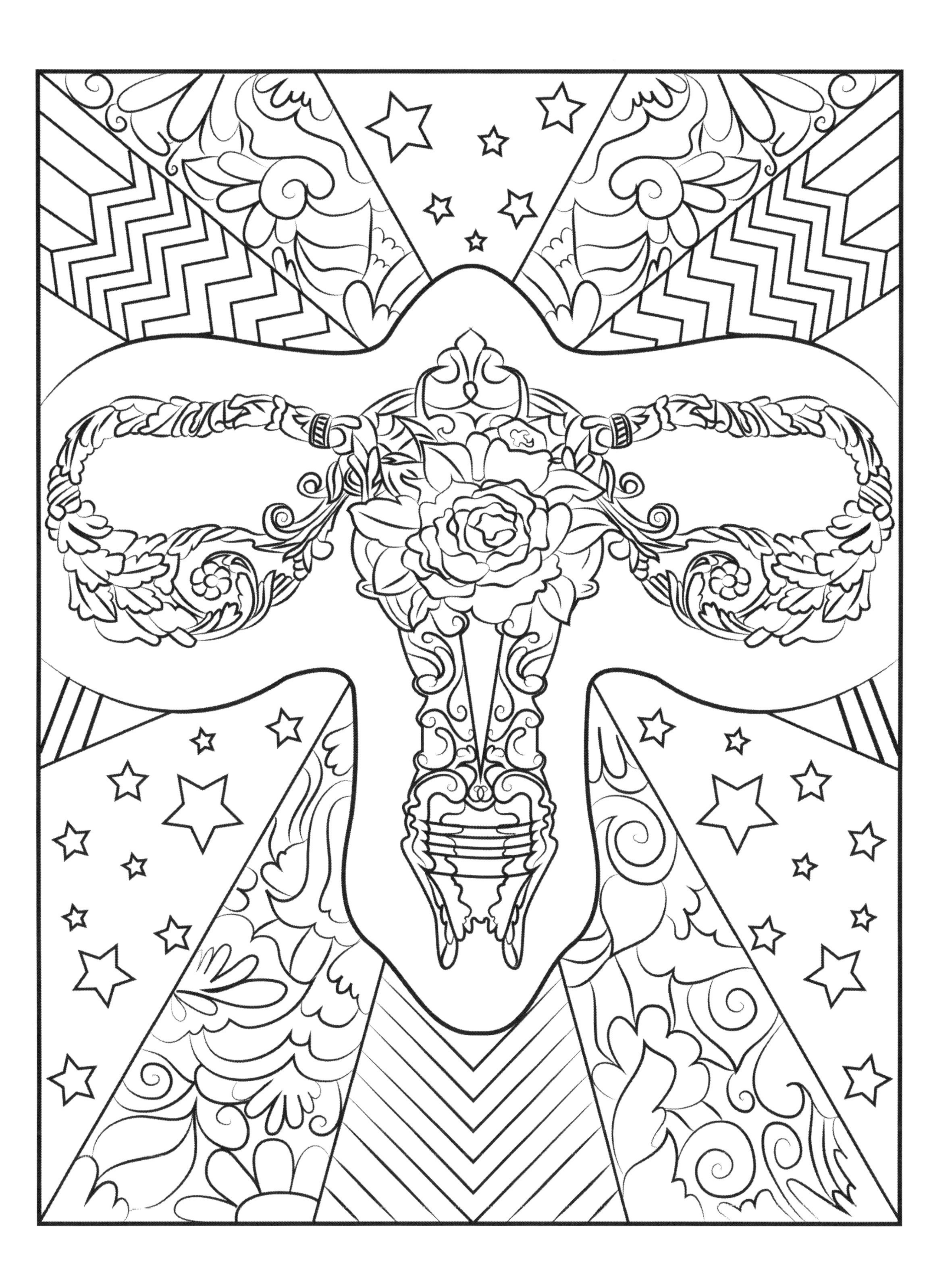

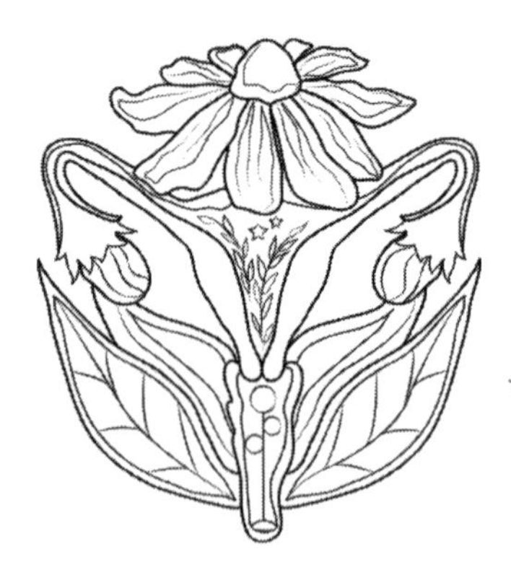

This page is intentionally left blank to avoid color bleeding.

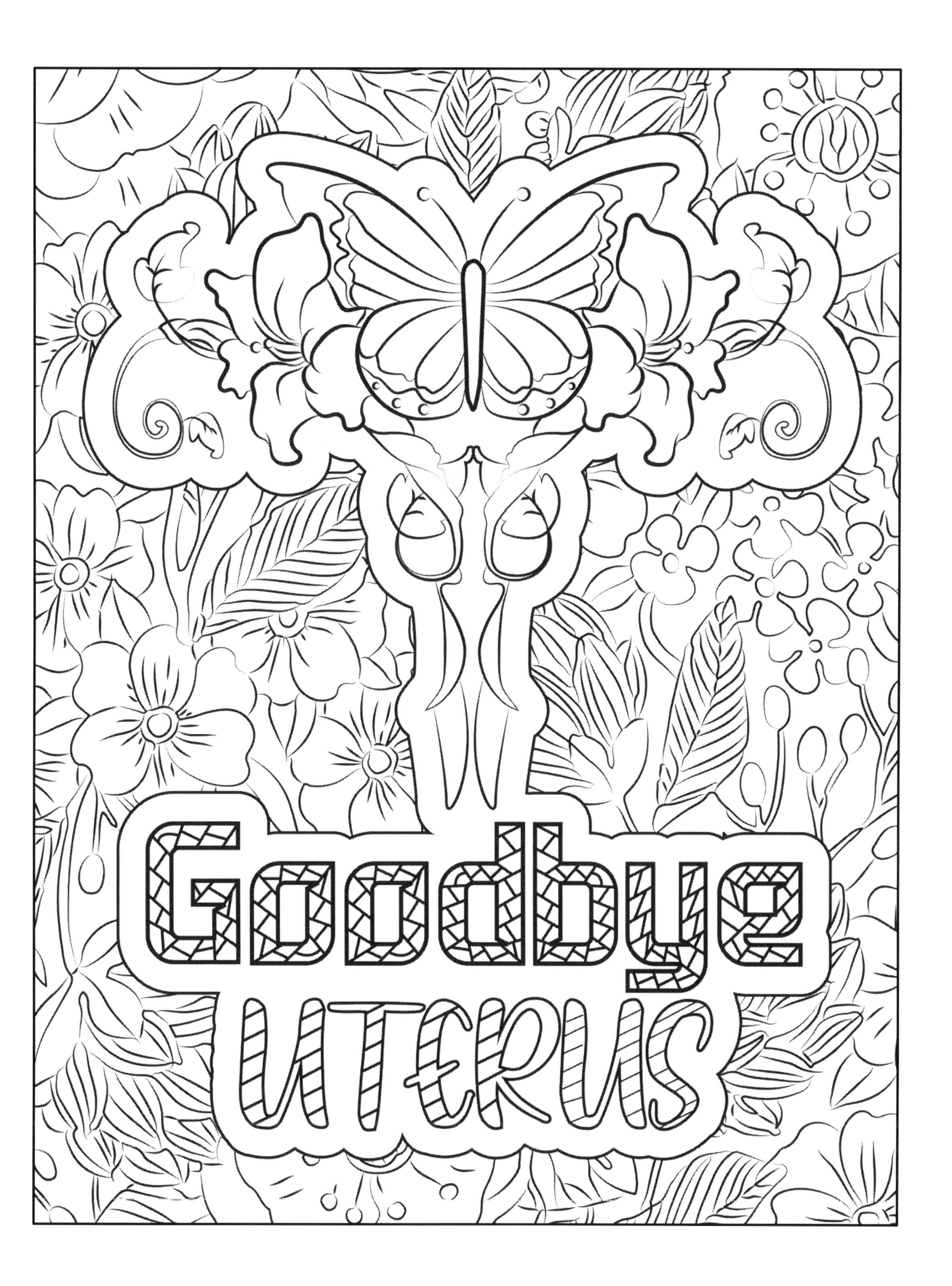
Goodbye
UTERUS

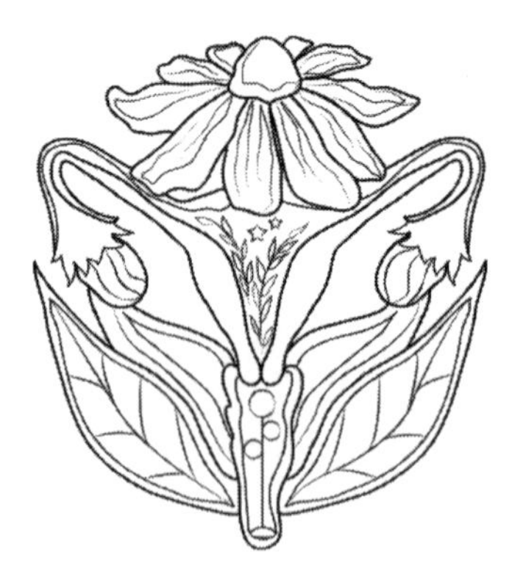

This page is intentionally left blank to avoid color bleeding.

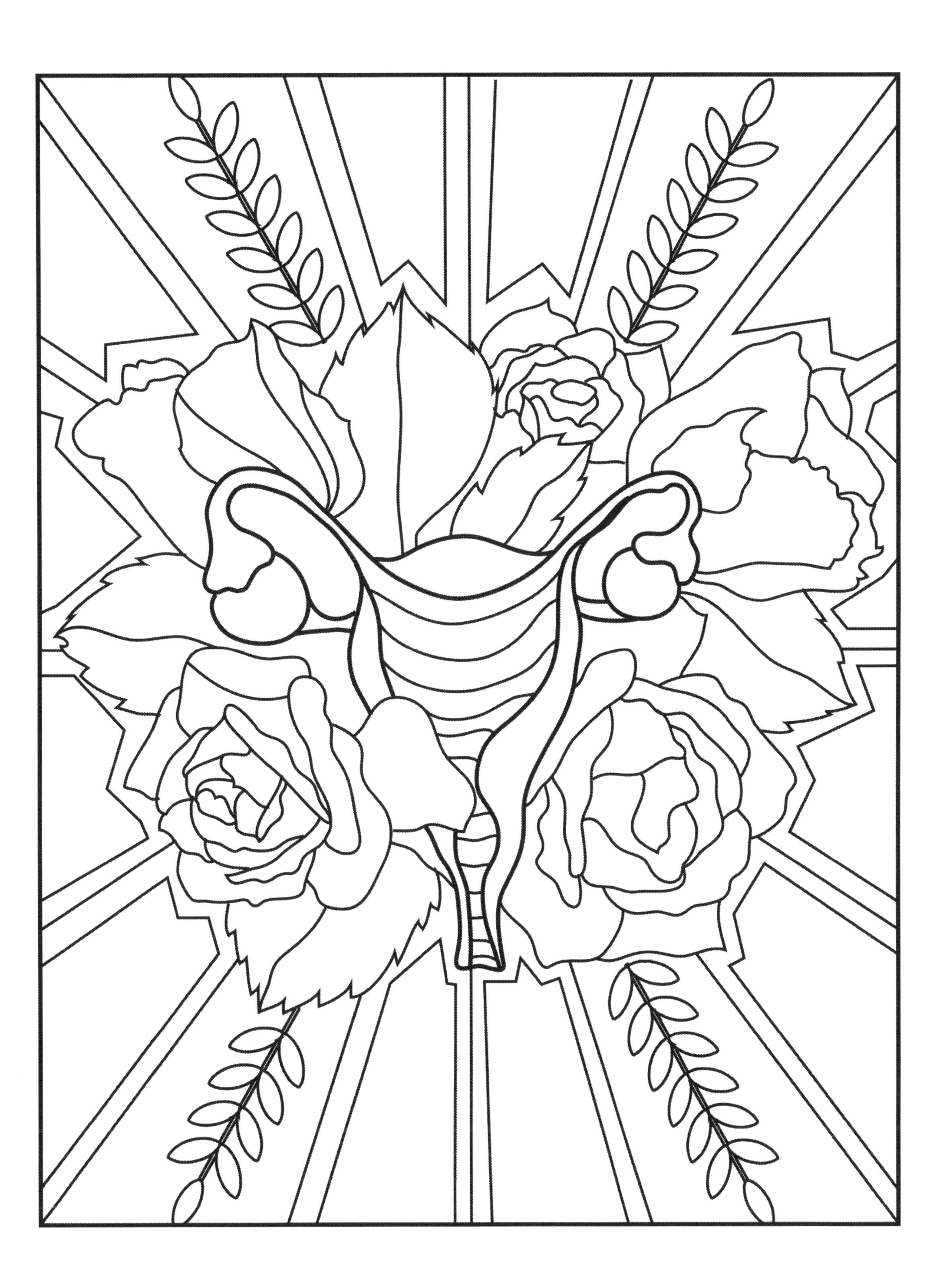

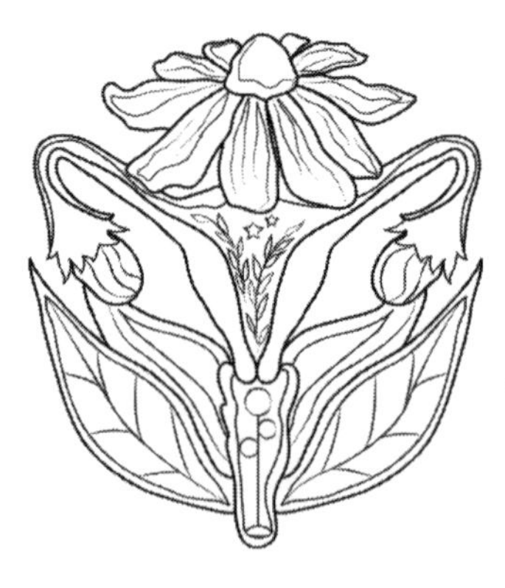

This page is intentionally left blank to avoid color bleeding.

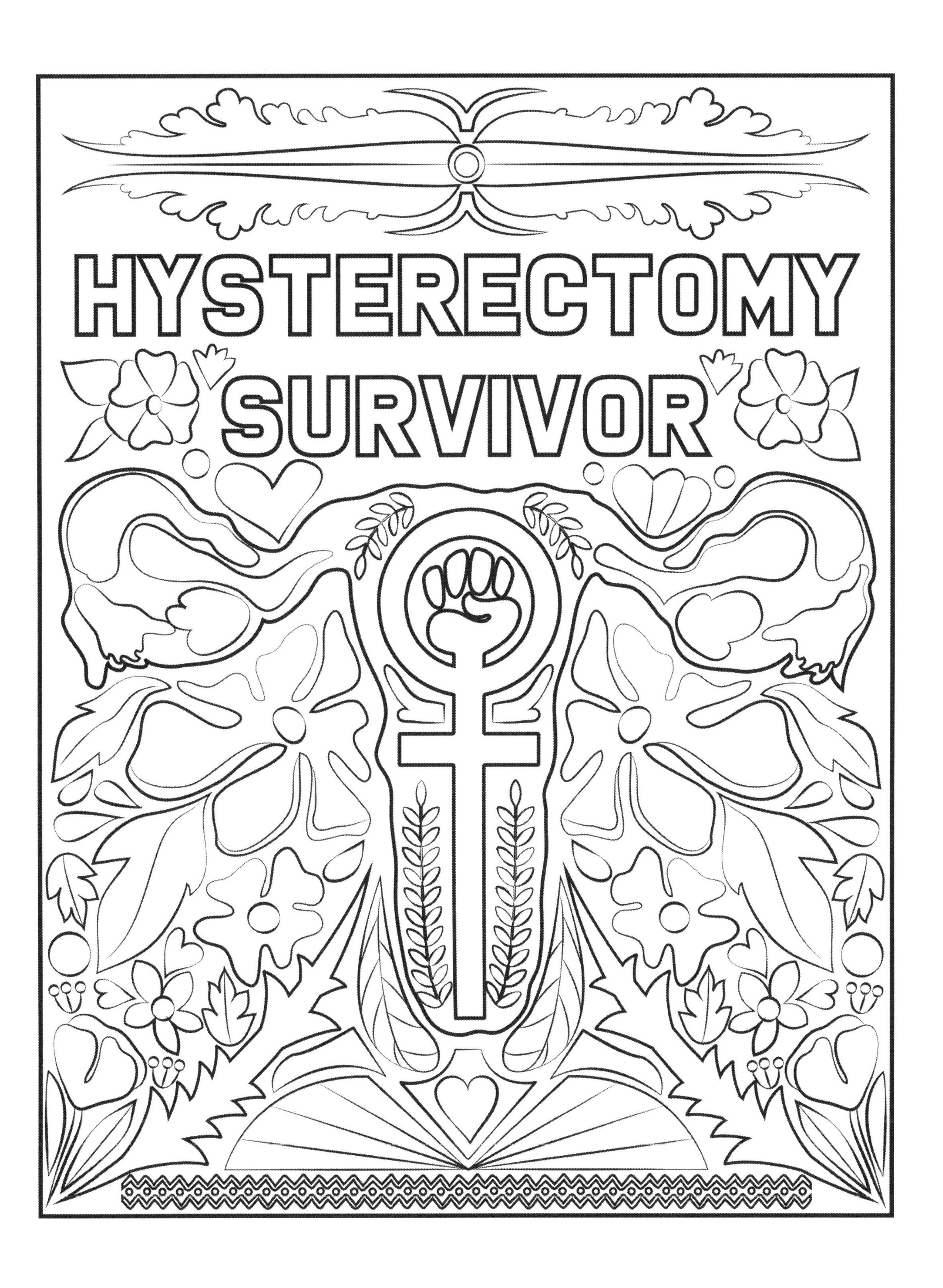
HYSTERECTOMY
SURVIVOR

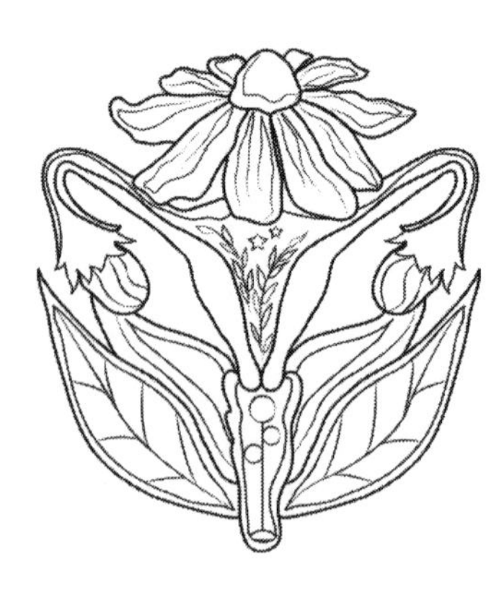

This page is intentionally left blank to avoid color bleeding.

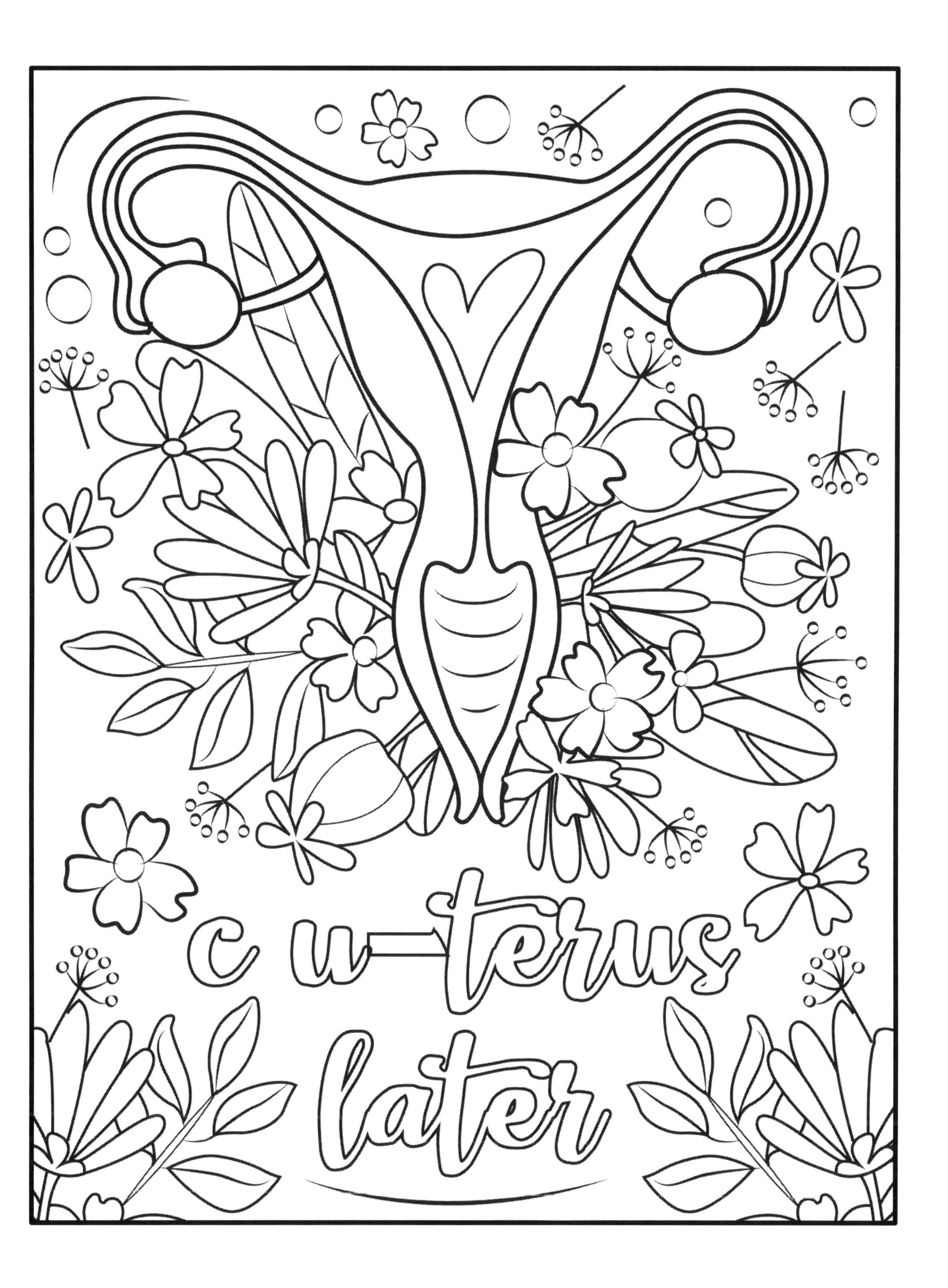
c u-terus
later

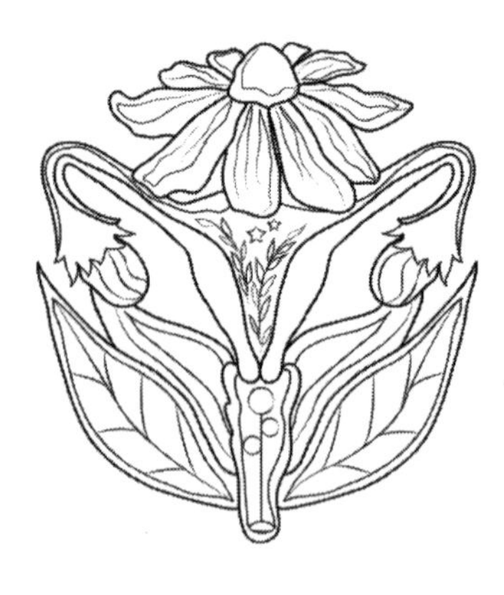

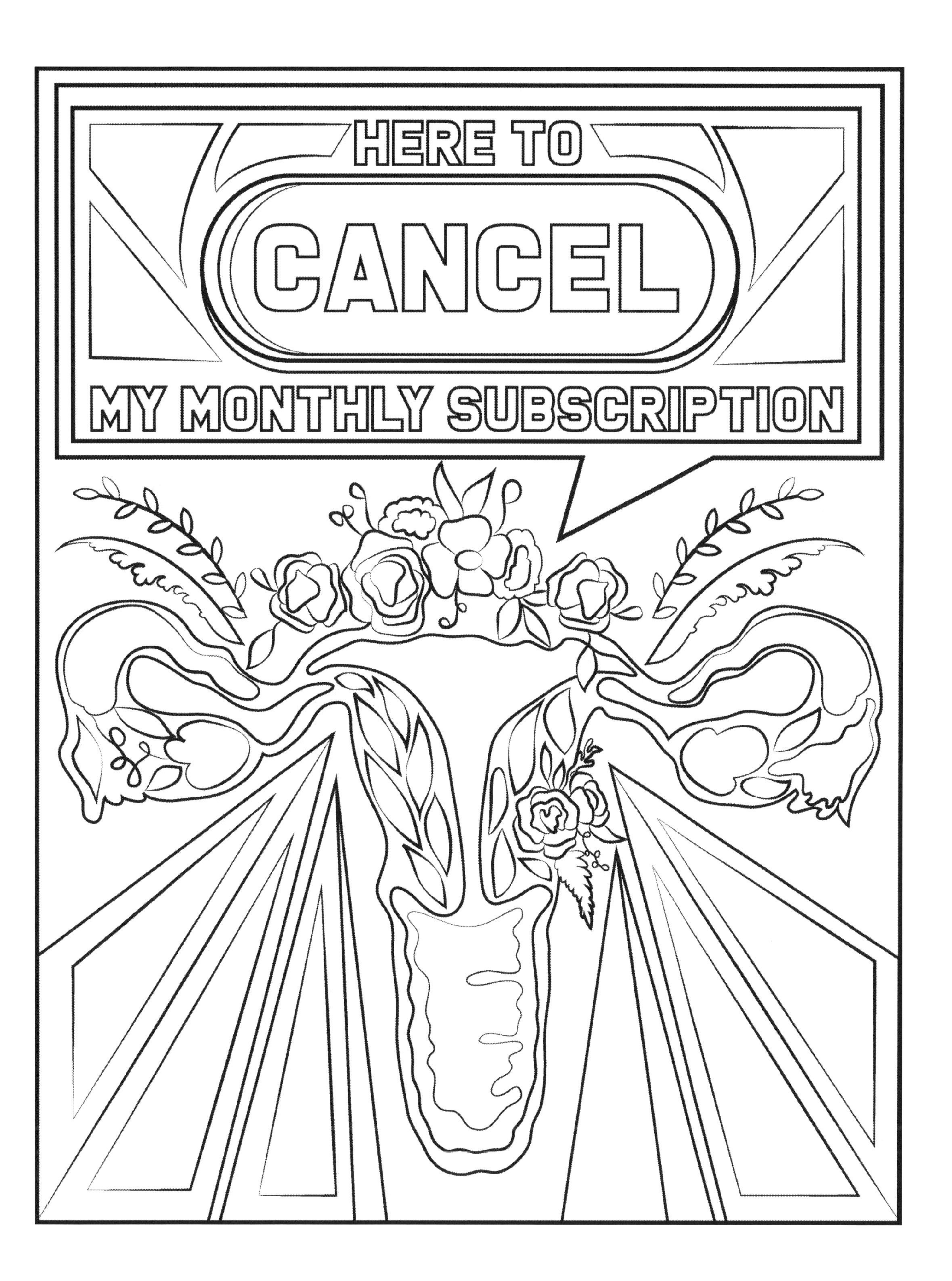
HERE TO
CANCEL
MY MONTHLY SUBSCRIPTION

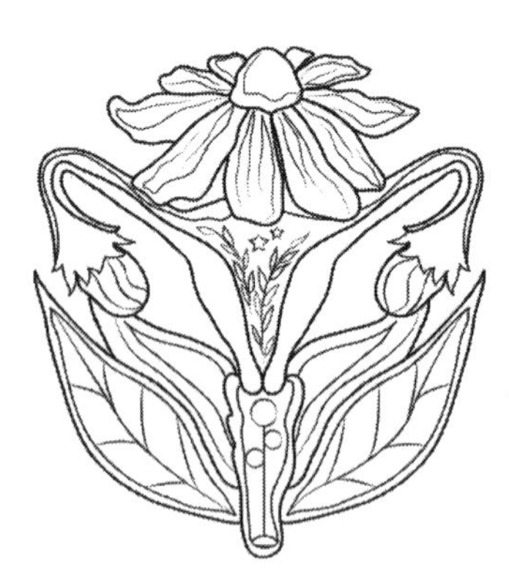

This page is intentionally left blank to avoid color bleeding.

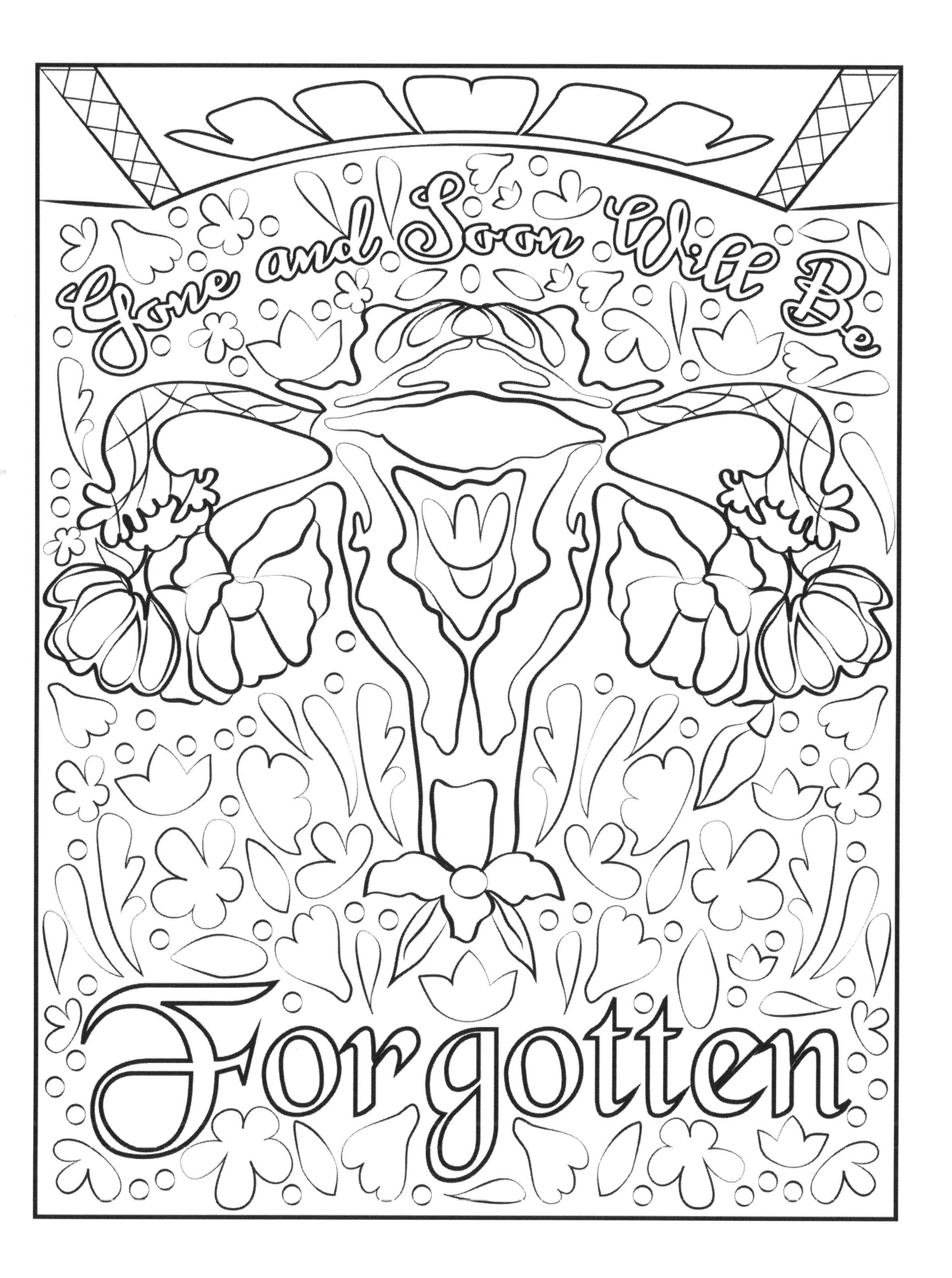
Gone and Soon Will Be
Forgotten

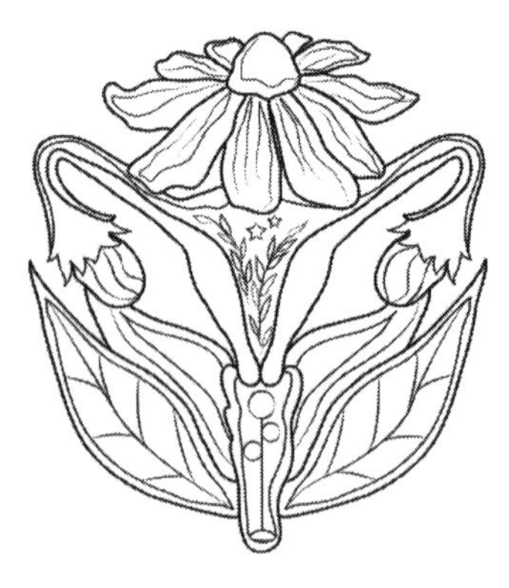

This page is intentionally left blank to avoid color bleeding.

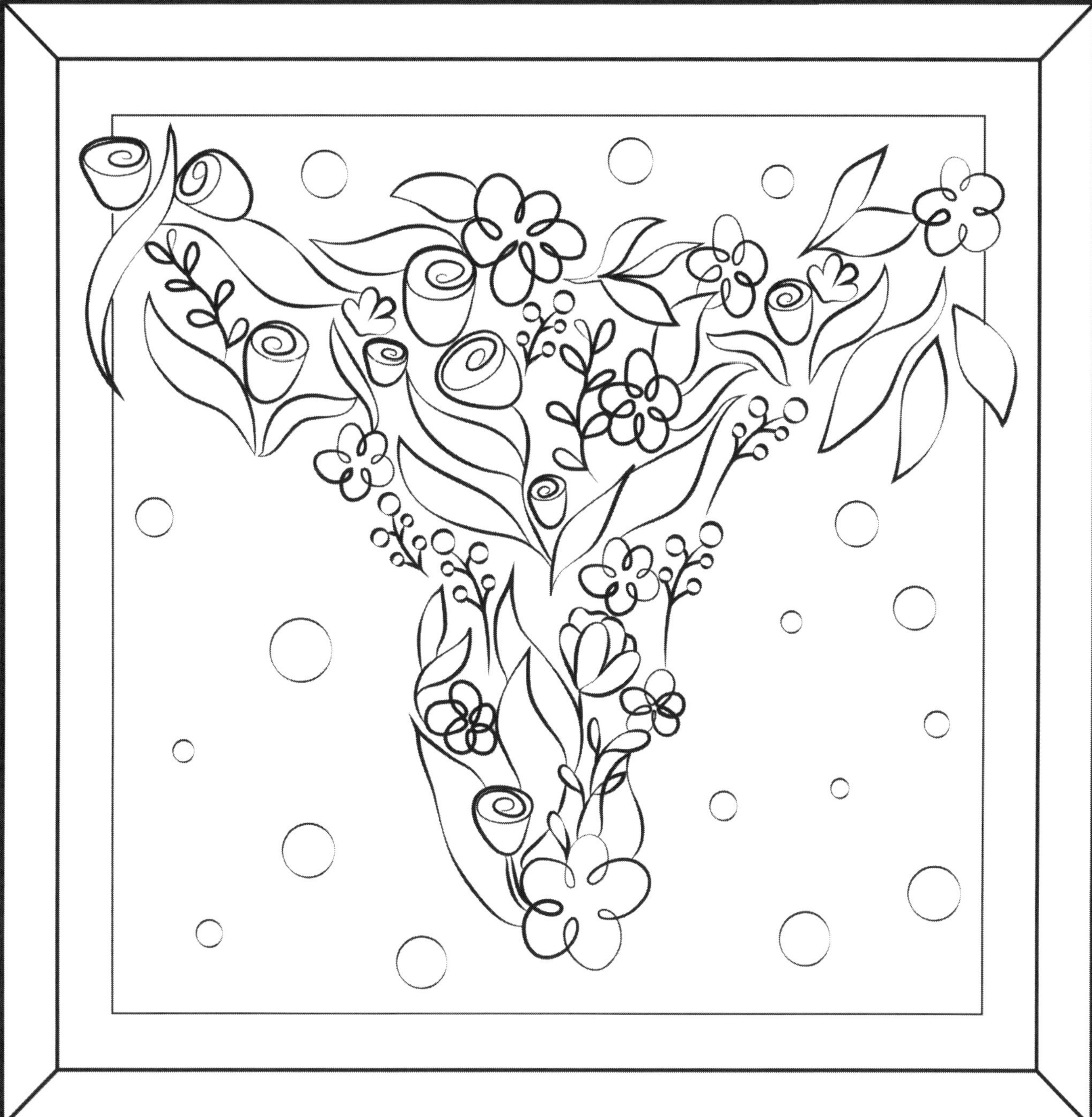

YOU'RE HYSTER-Y,
I'M SO OVARY YOU

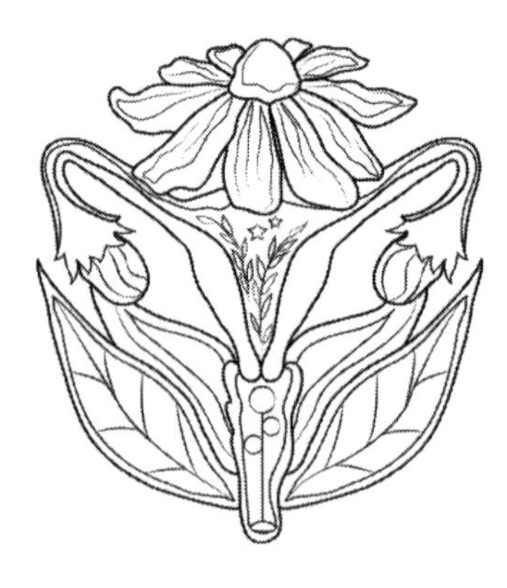

This page is intentionally left blank to avoid color bleeding.

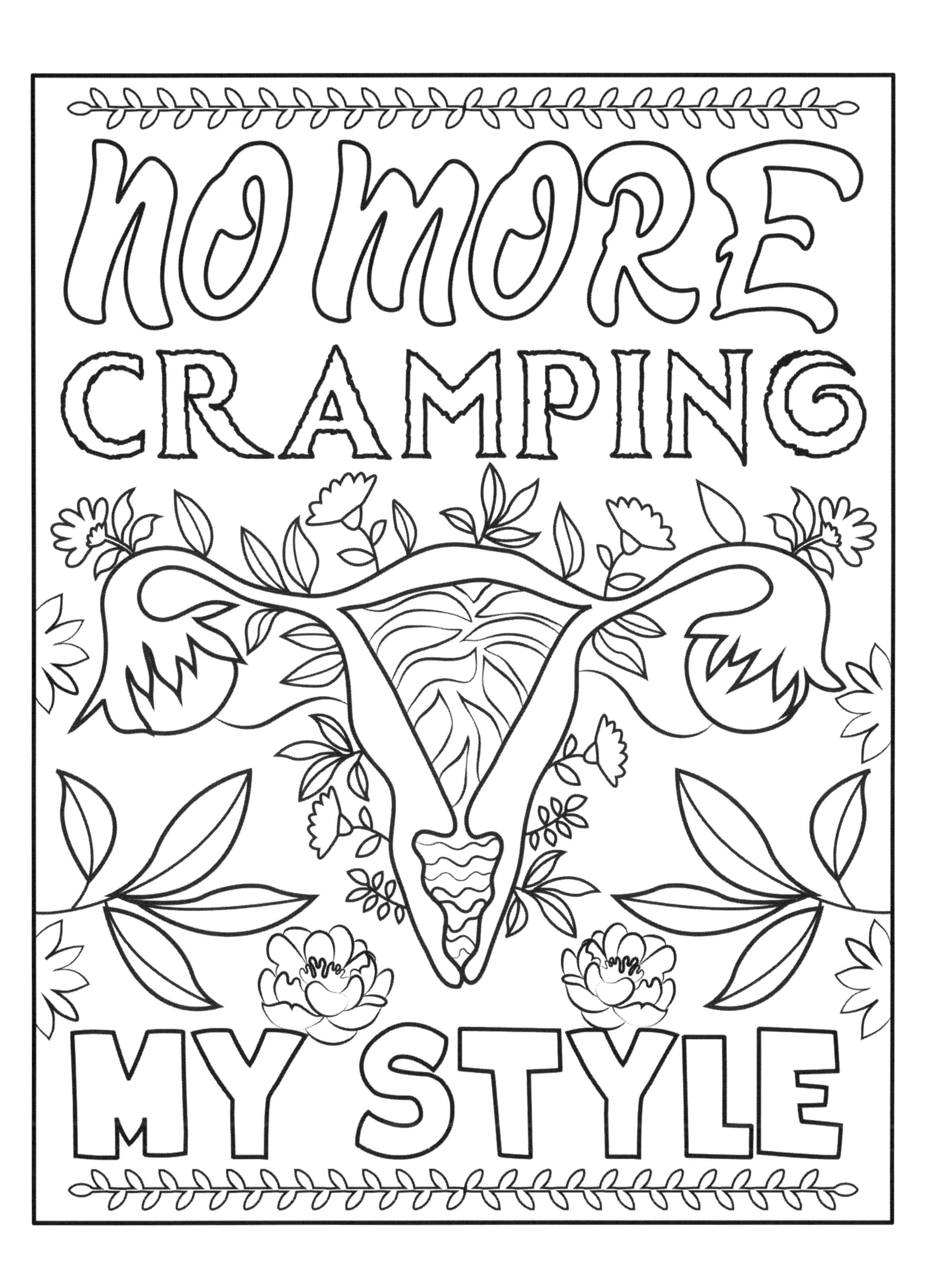
NO MORE
CRAMPING
MY STYLE

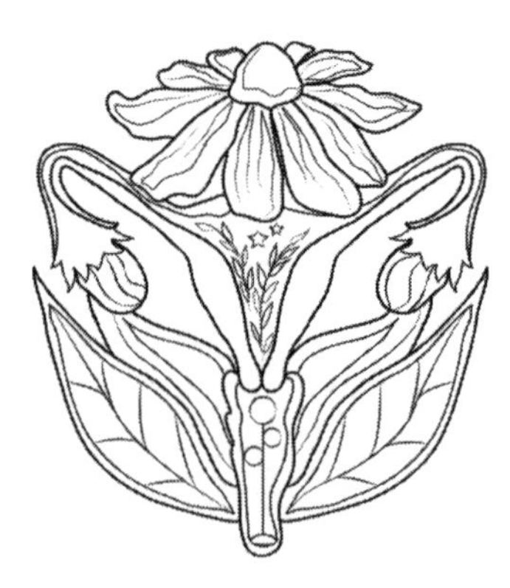

This page is intentionally left blank to avoid color bleeding.

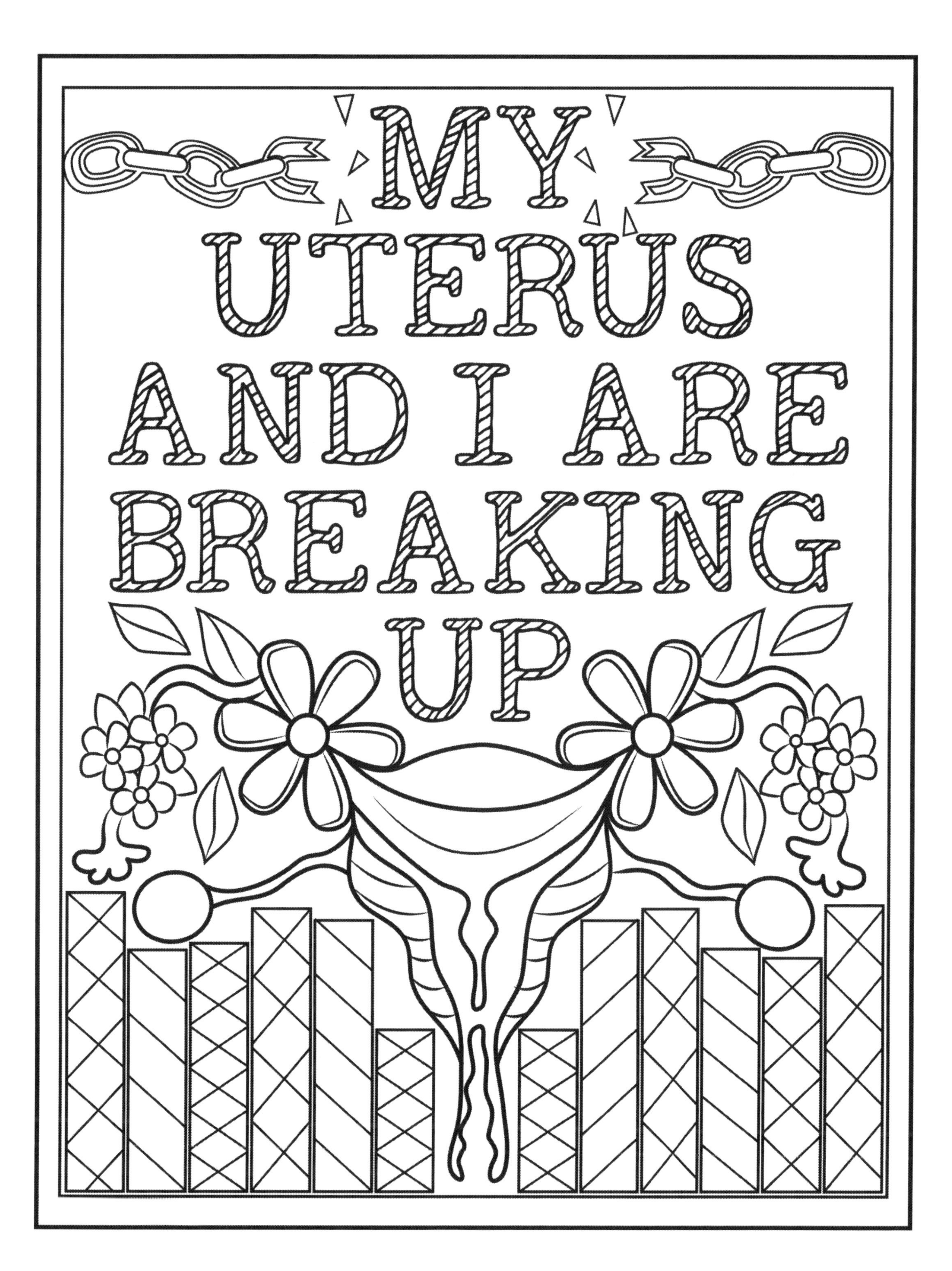
MY
UTERUS
AND I ARE
BREAKING
UP

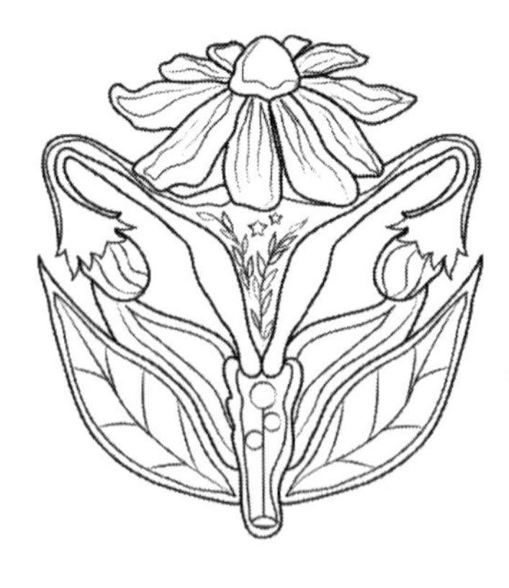

This page is intentionally left blank to avoid color bleeding.

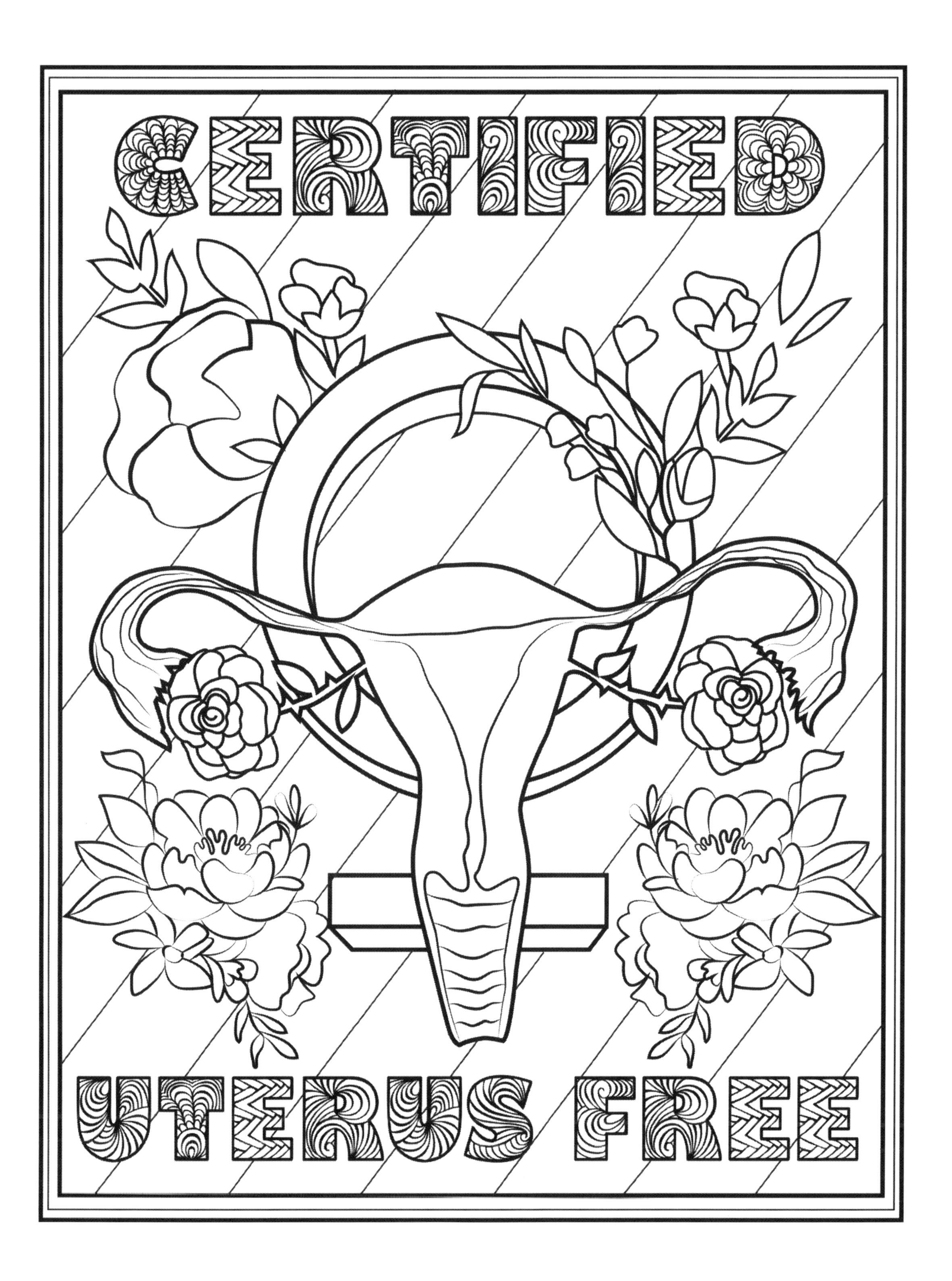
CERTIFIED
UTERUS FREE

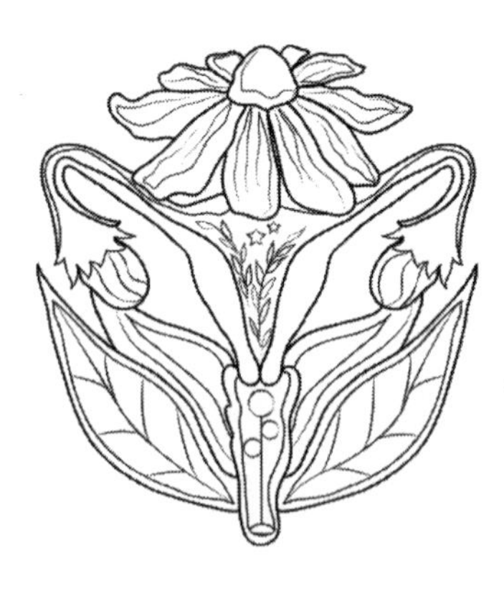

This page is intentionally left blank to avoid color bleeding.

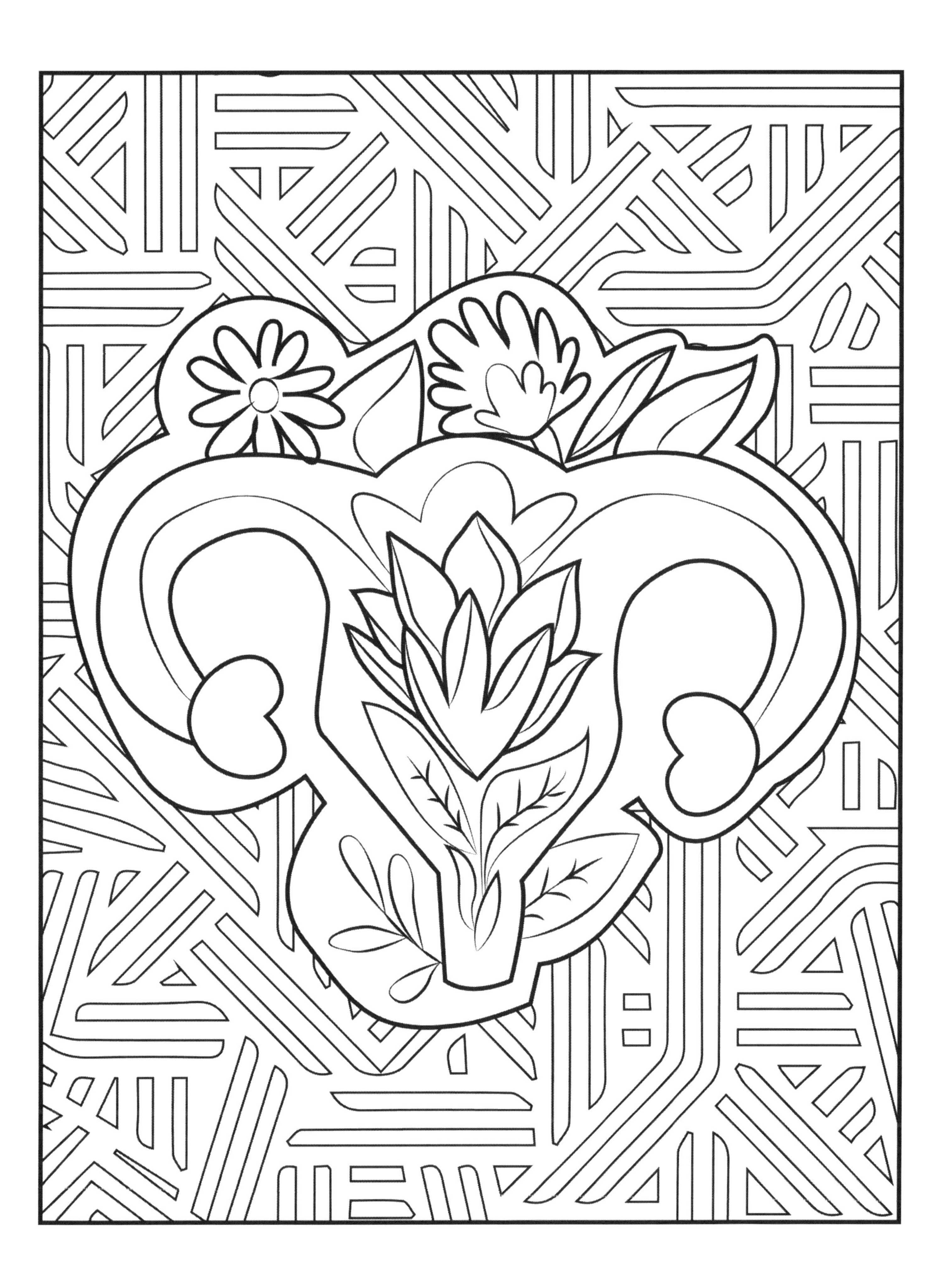

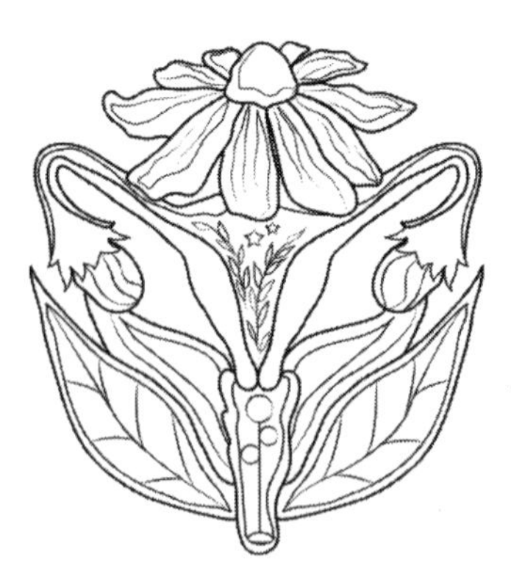

This page is intentionally left blank to avoid color bleeding.

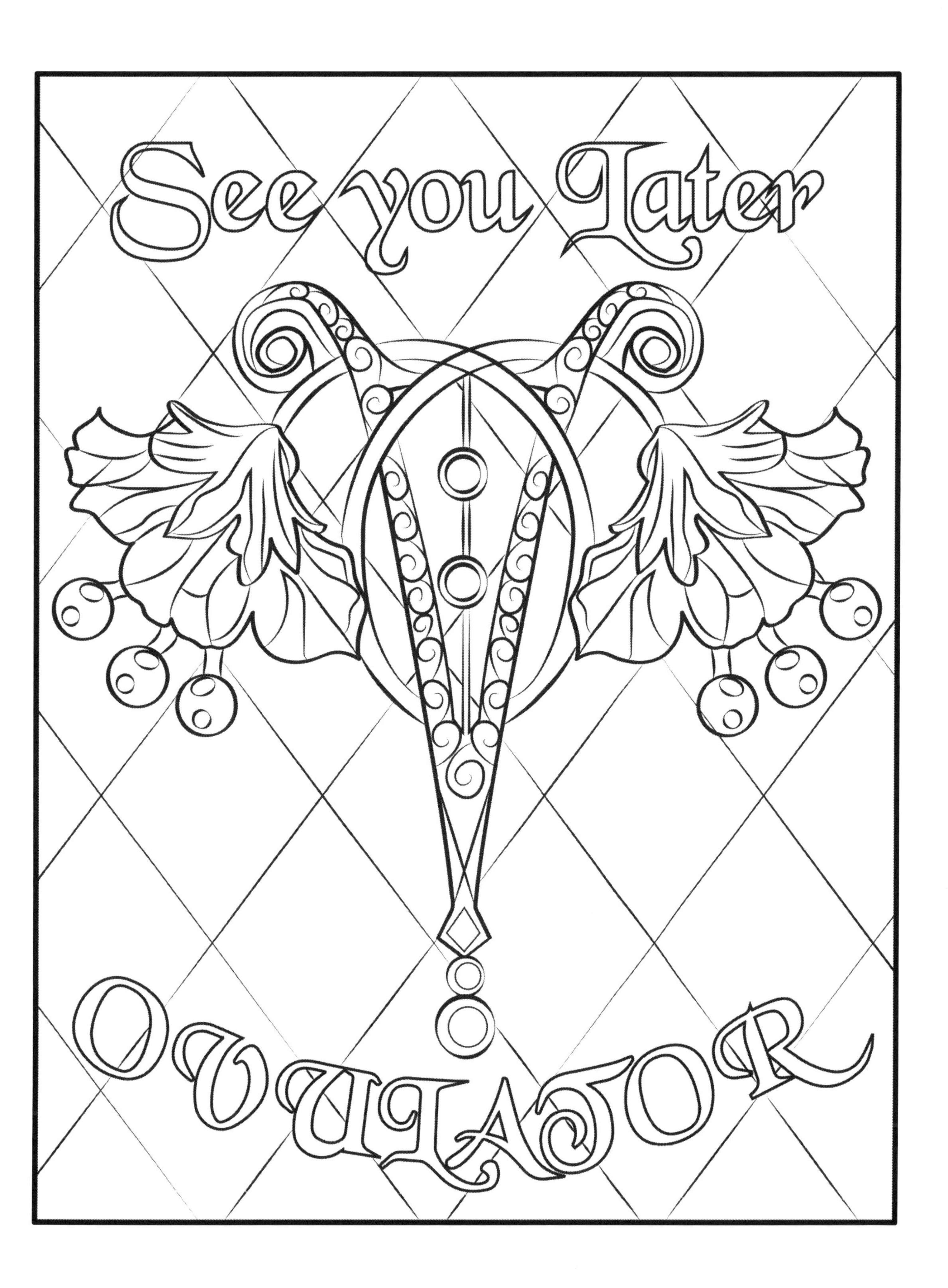
See you Later
OVULATOR

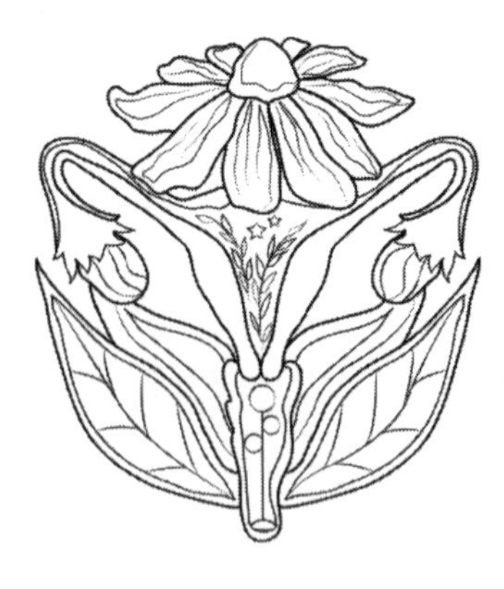

This page is intentionally left blank to avoid color bleeding.

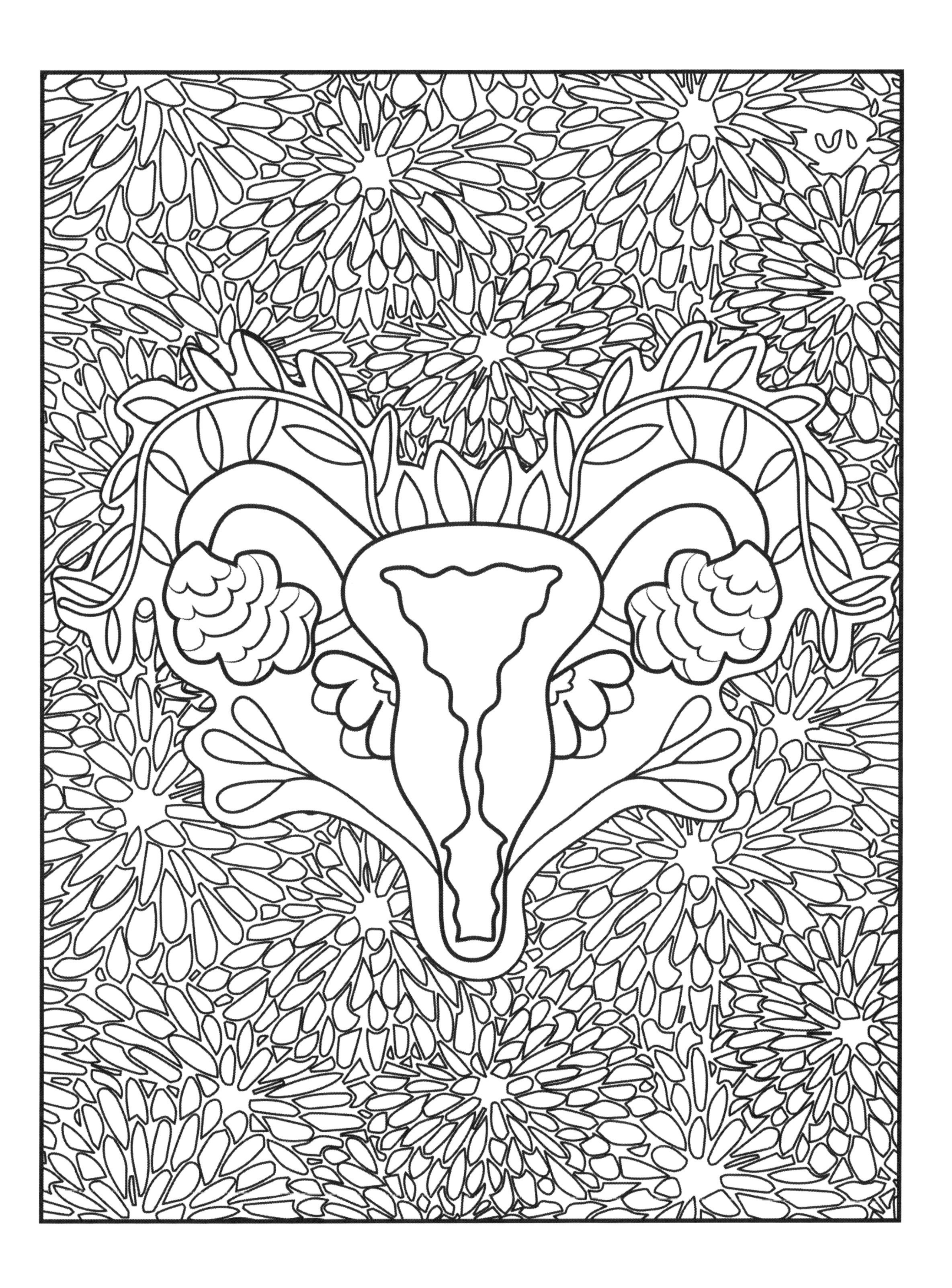

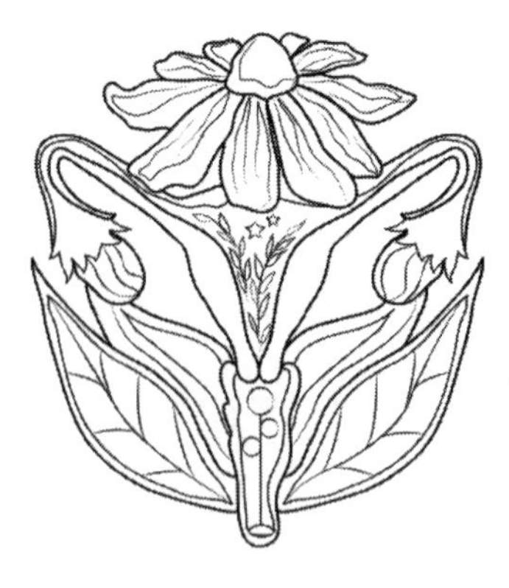

This page is intentionally left blank to avoid color bleeding.

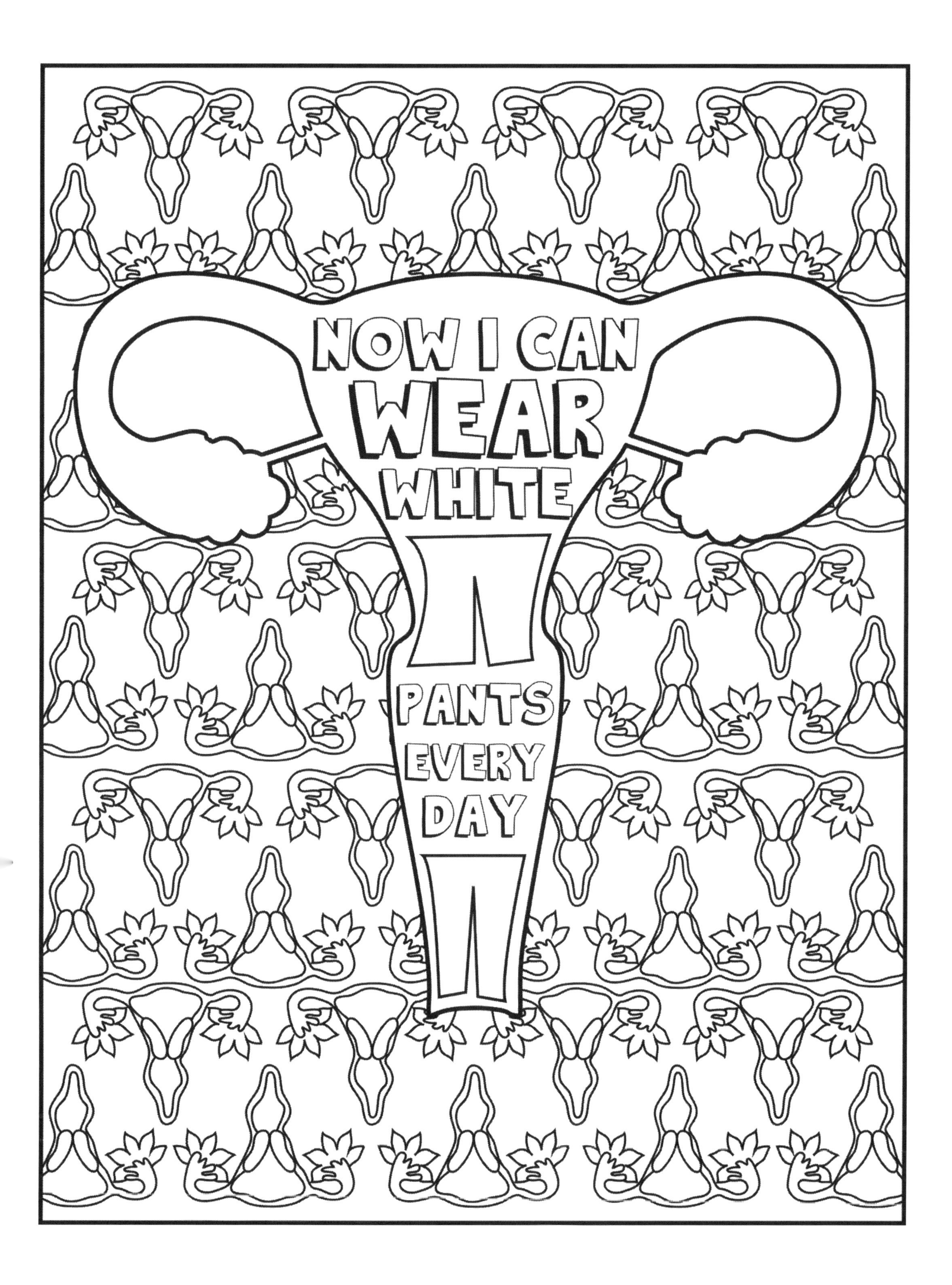
NOW I CAN
WEAR
WHITE
PANTS
EVERY
DAY

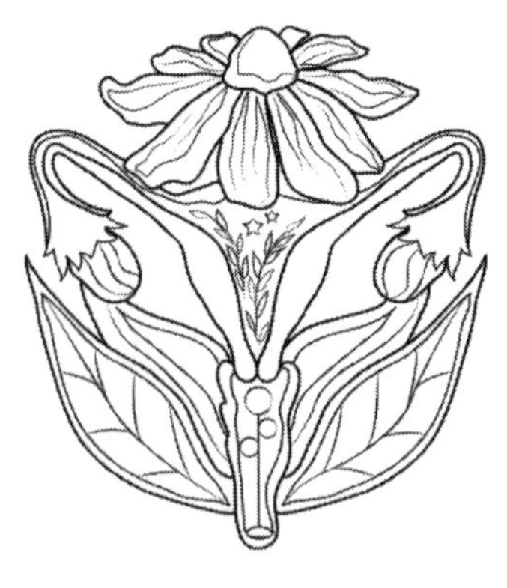

This page is intentionally left blank to avoid color bleeding.

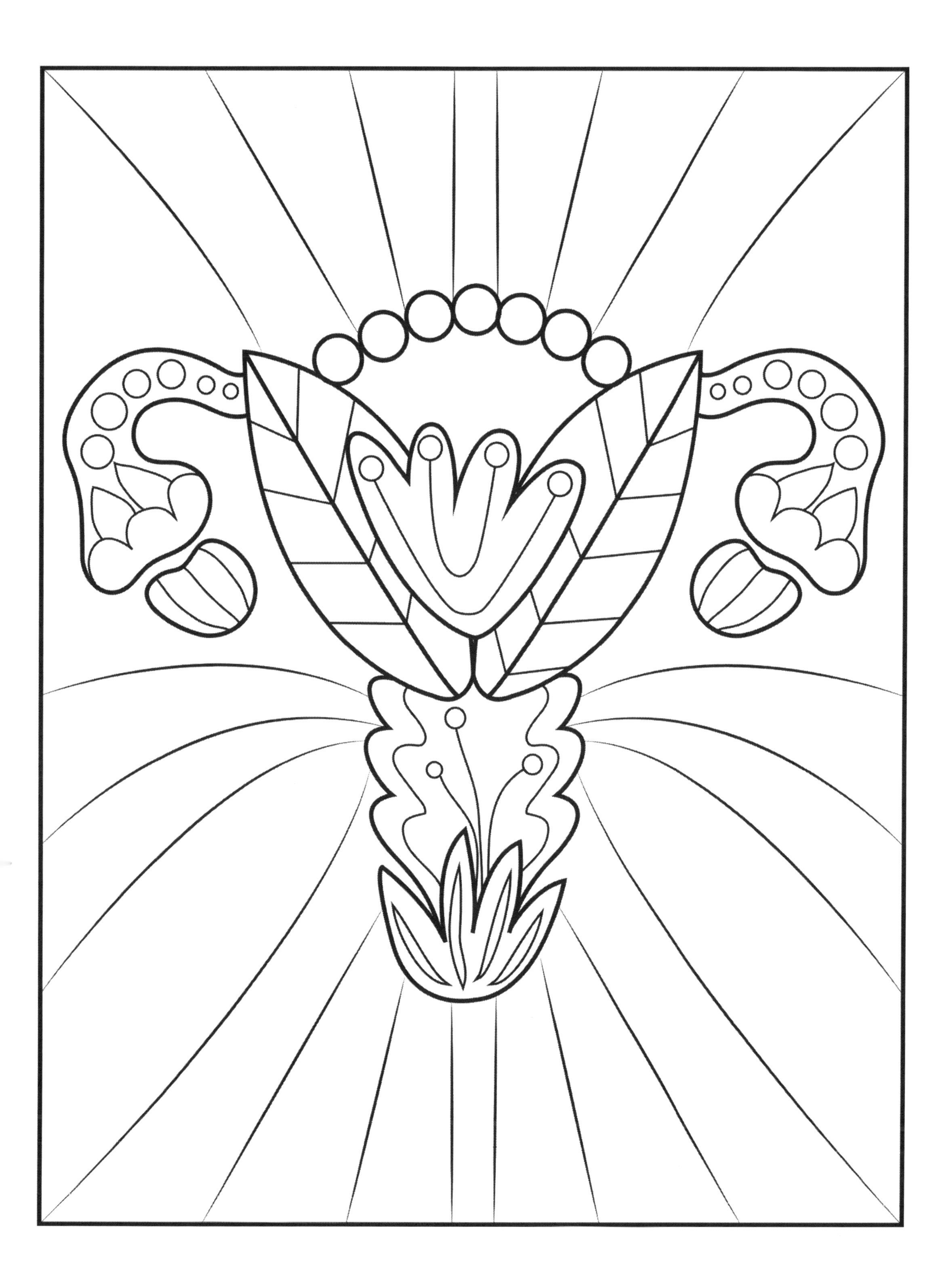

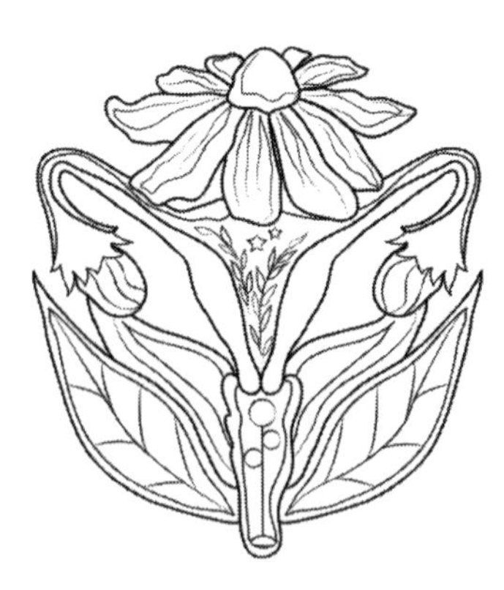

This page is intentionally left blank to avoid color bleeding.

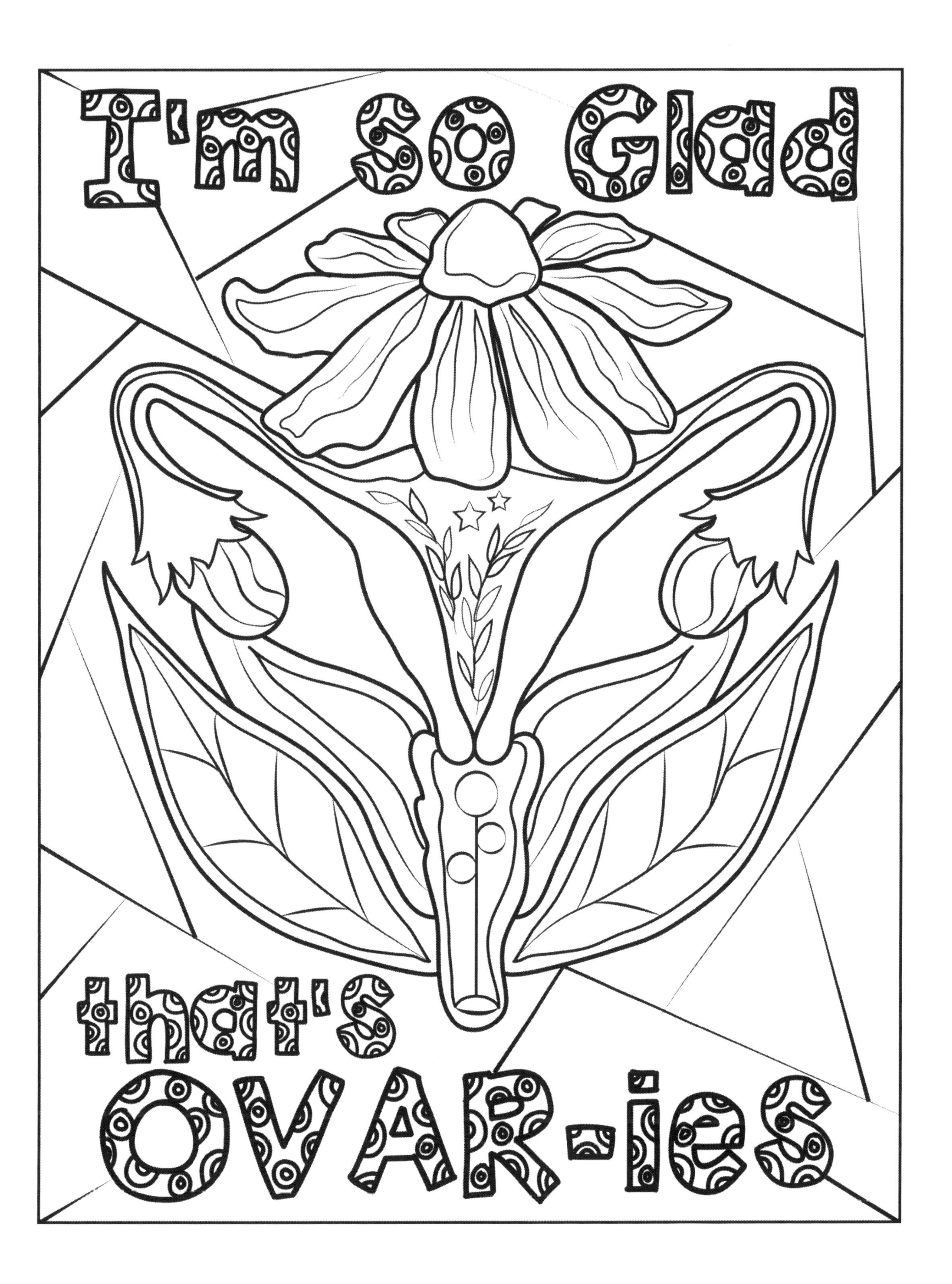
I'm so Glad
that's
OVAR-ies

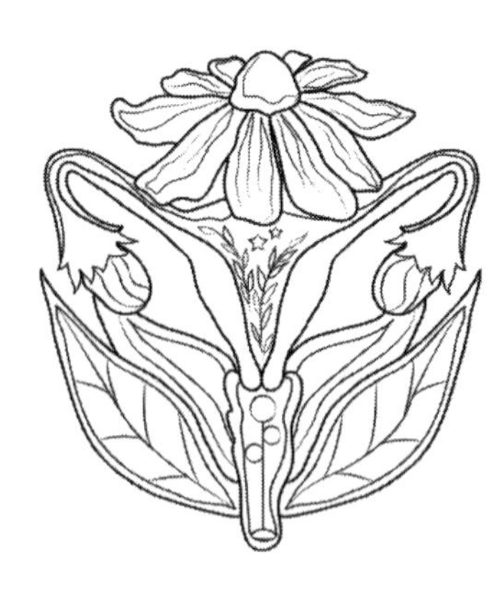

This page is intentionally left blank to avoid color bleeding.

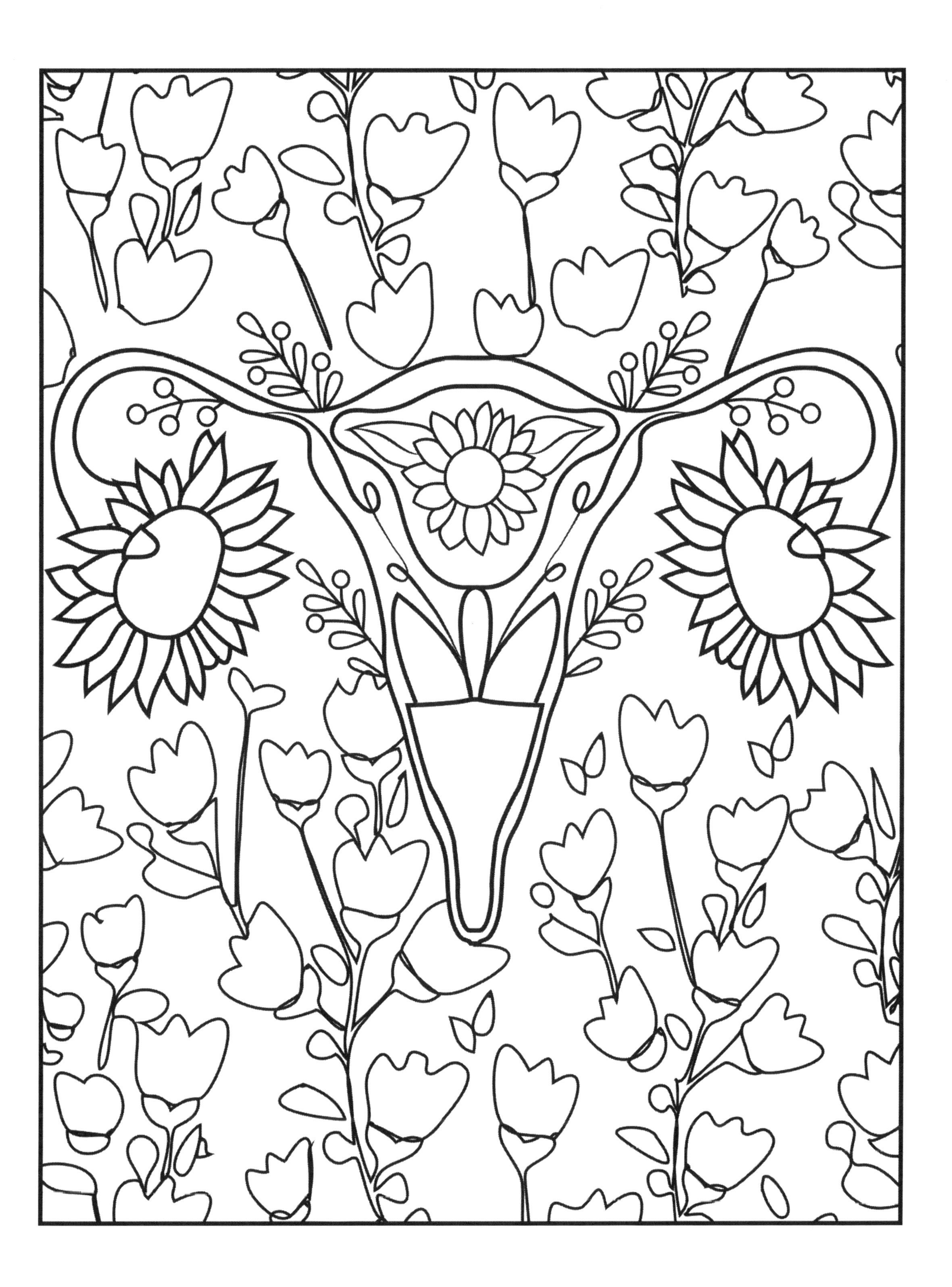

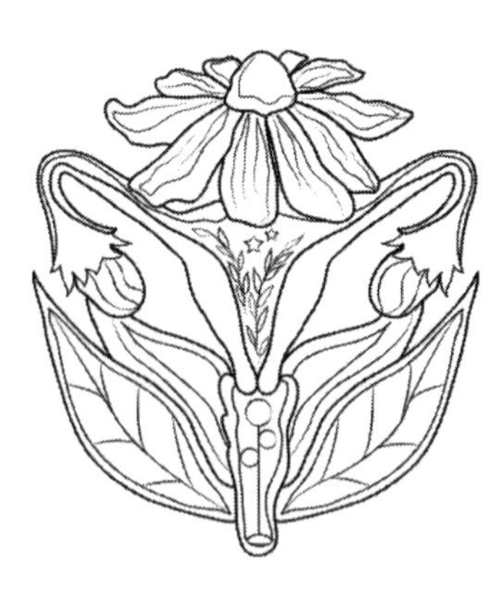

This page is intentionally left blank to avoid color bleeding.

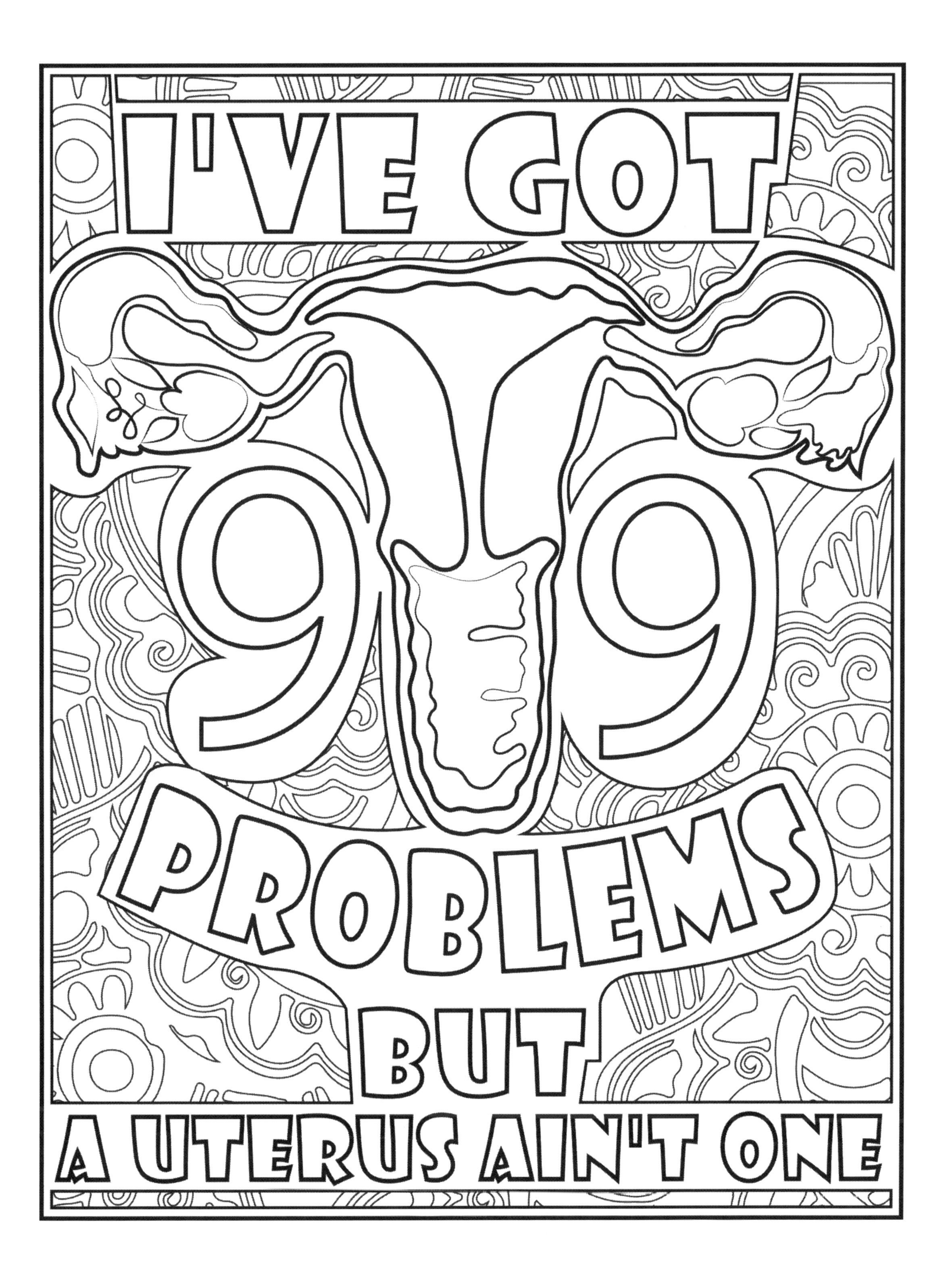
I'VE GOT
99
PROBLEMS
BUT
A UTERUS AIN'T ONE

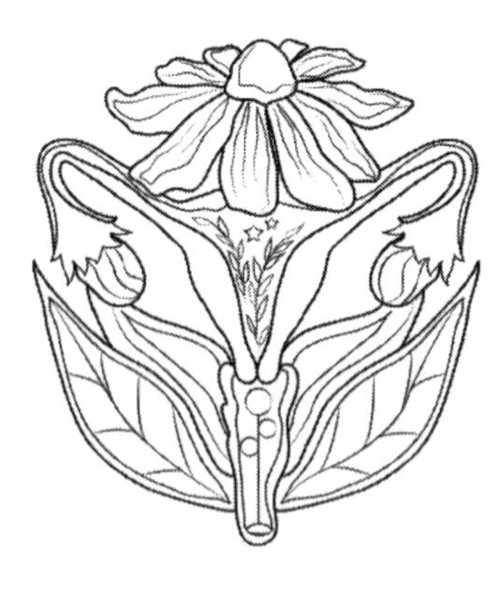

This page is intentionally left blank to avoid color bleeding.

Monthly subscription canceled

I'm so glad that's

OVAR-ies

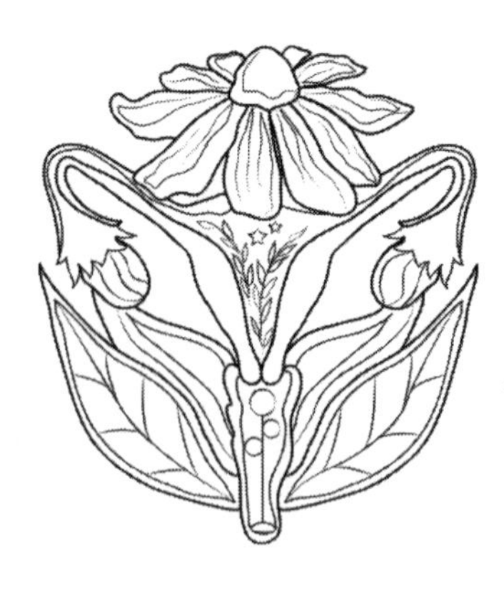

This page is intentionally left blank to avoid color bleeding.

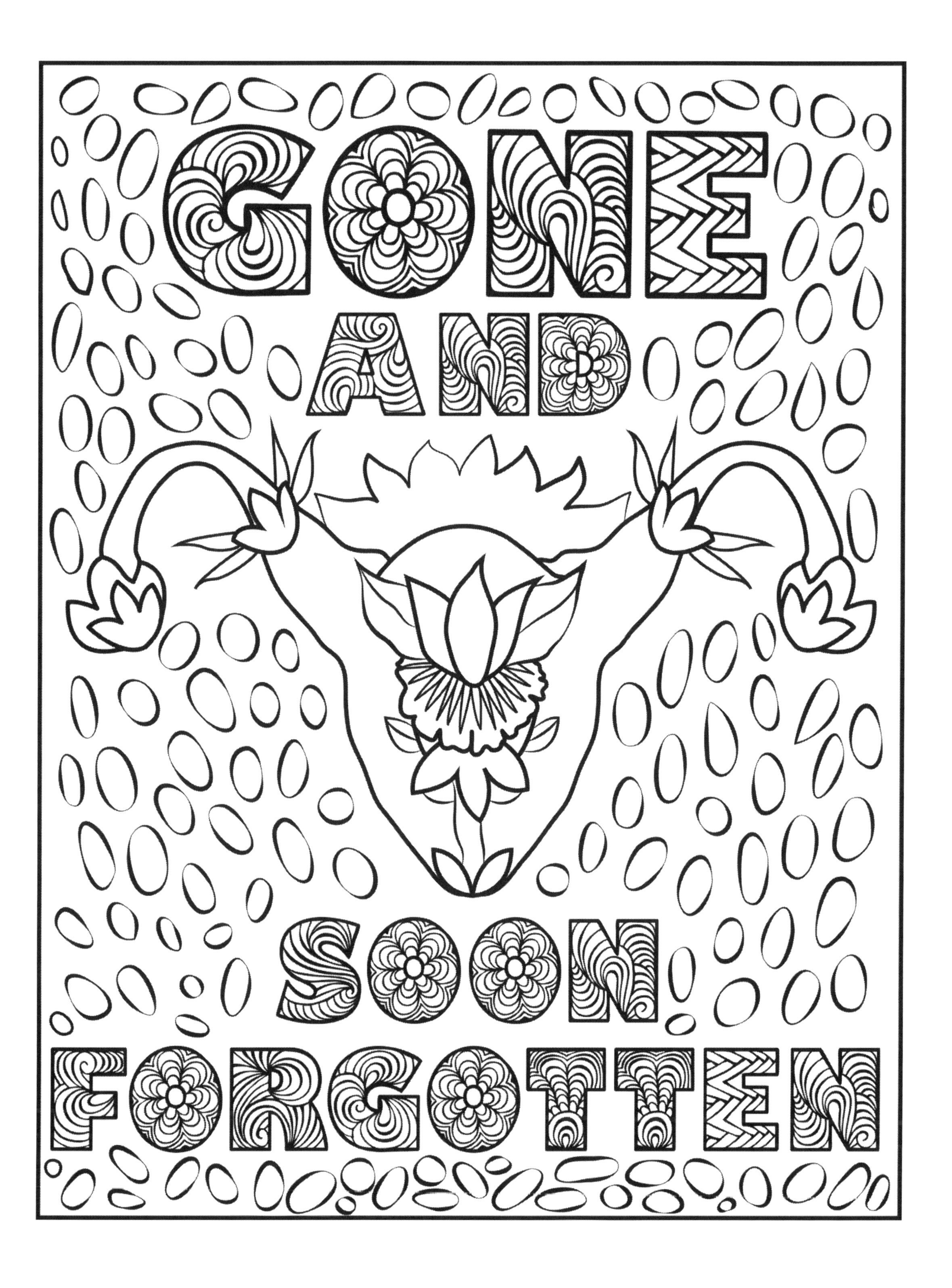
GONE
AND
SOON
FORGOTTEN

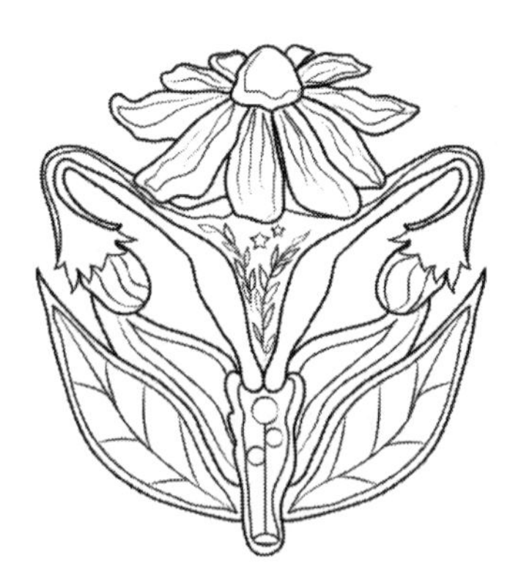

This page is intentionally left blank to avoid color bleeding.

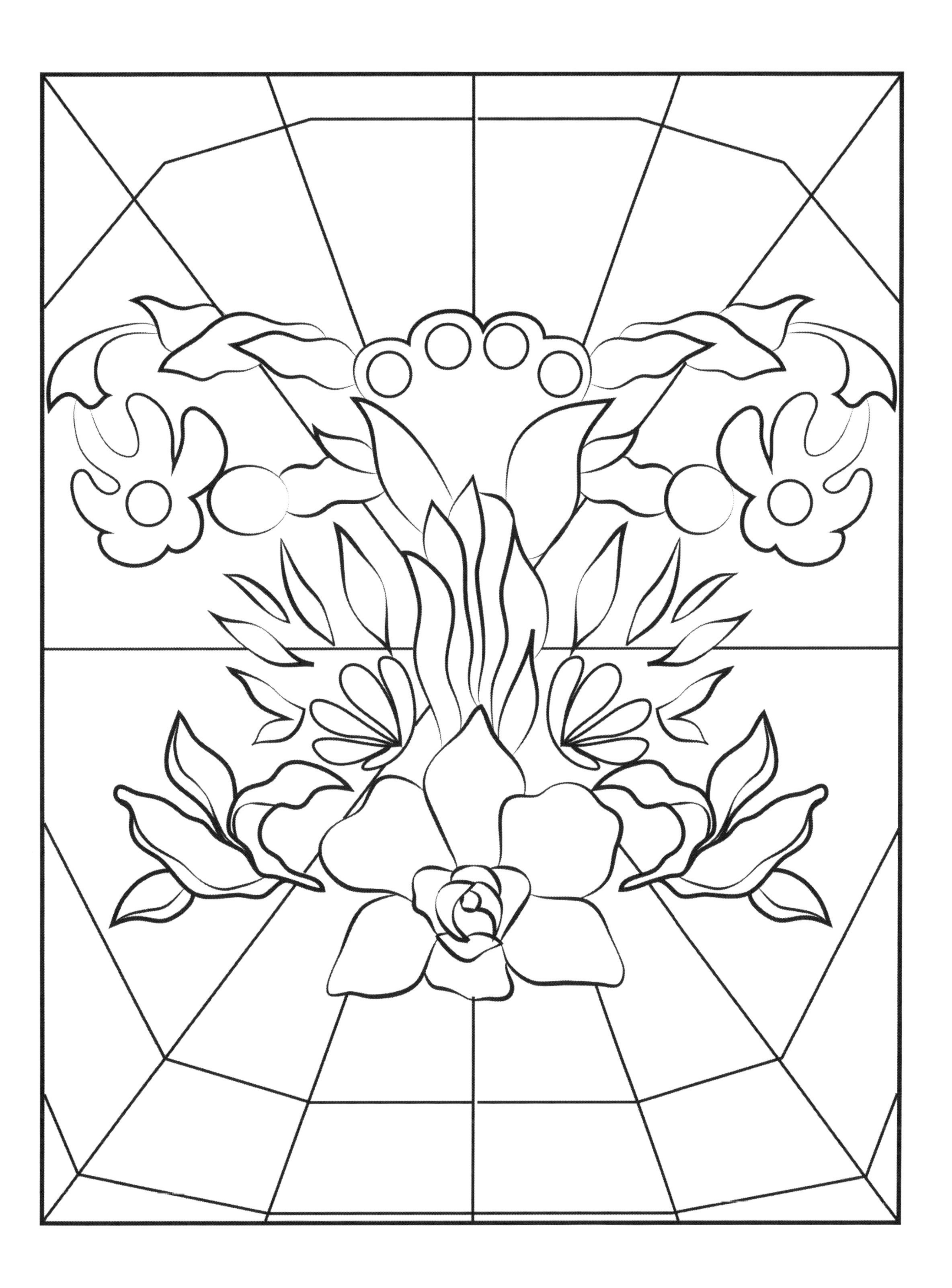

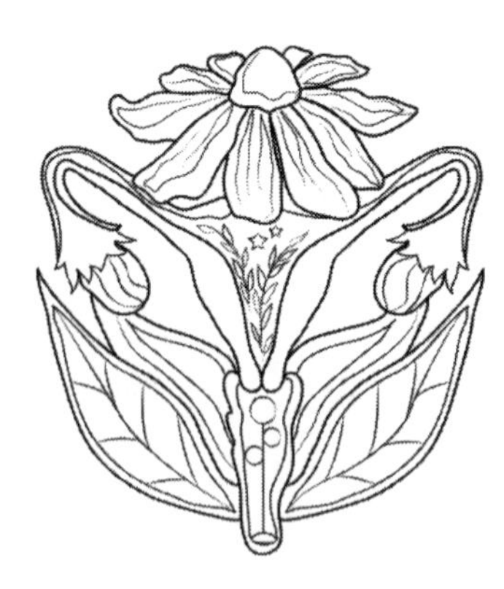

This page is intentionally left blank to avoid color bleeding.

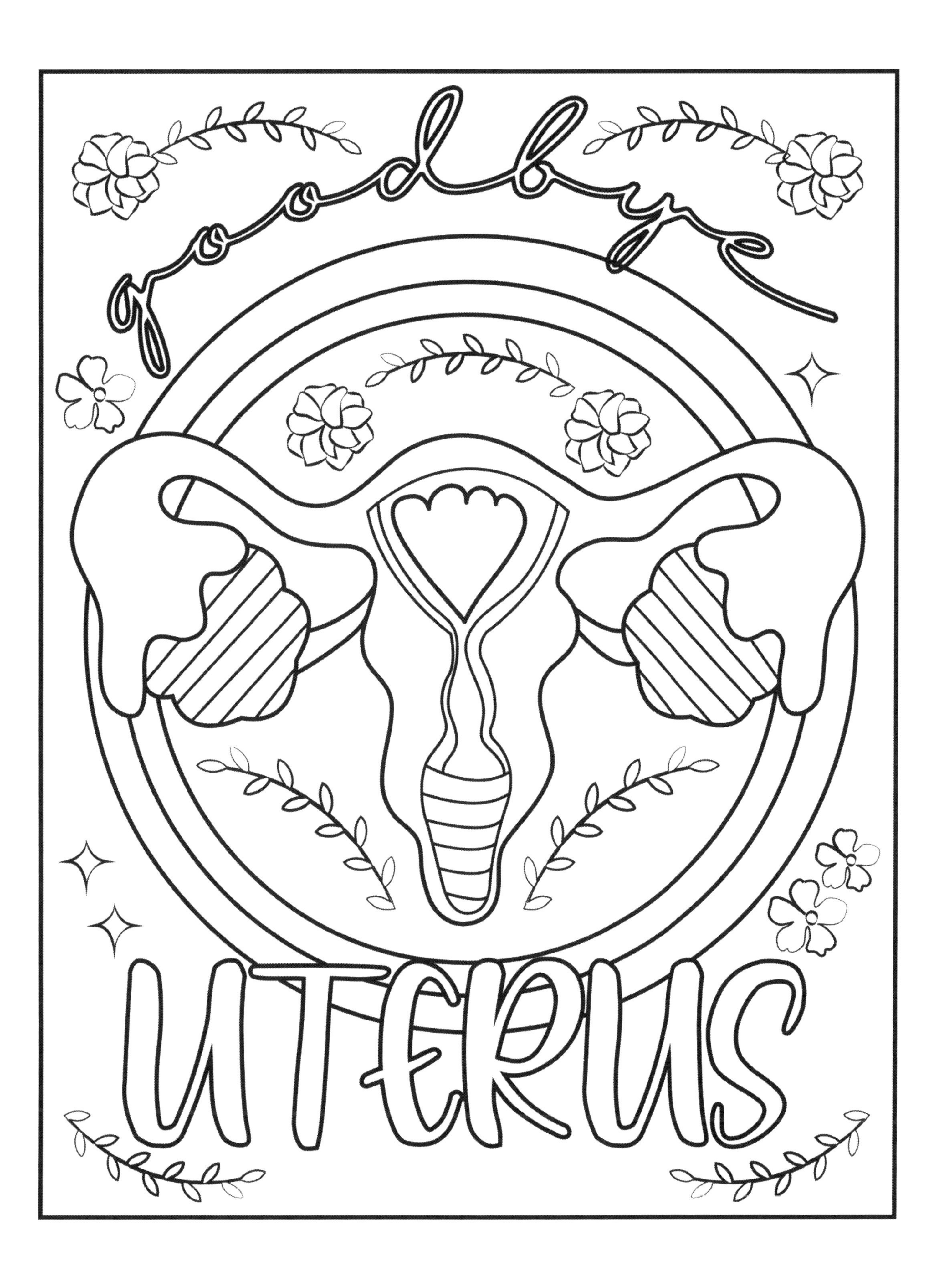
goodbye
UTERUS

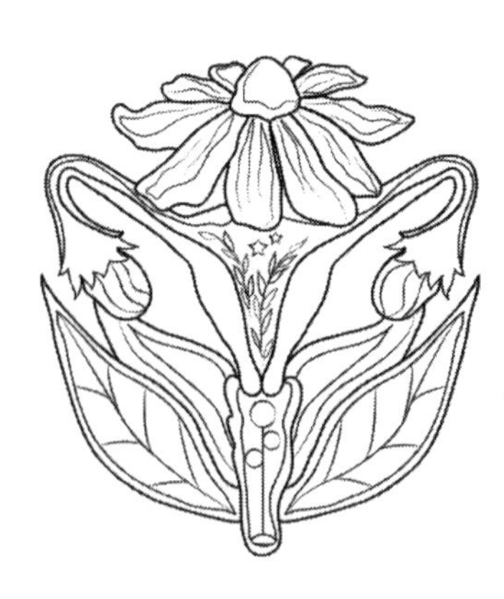

This page is intentionally left blank to avoid color bleeding.

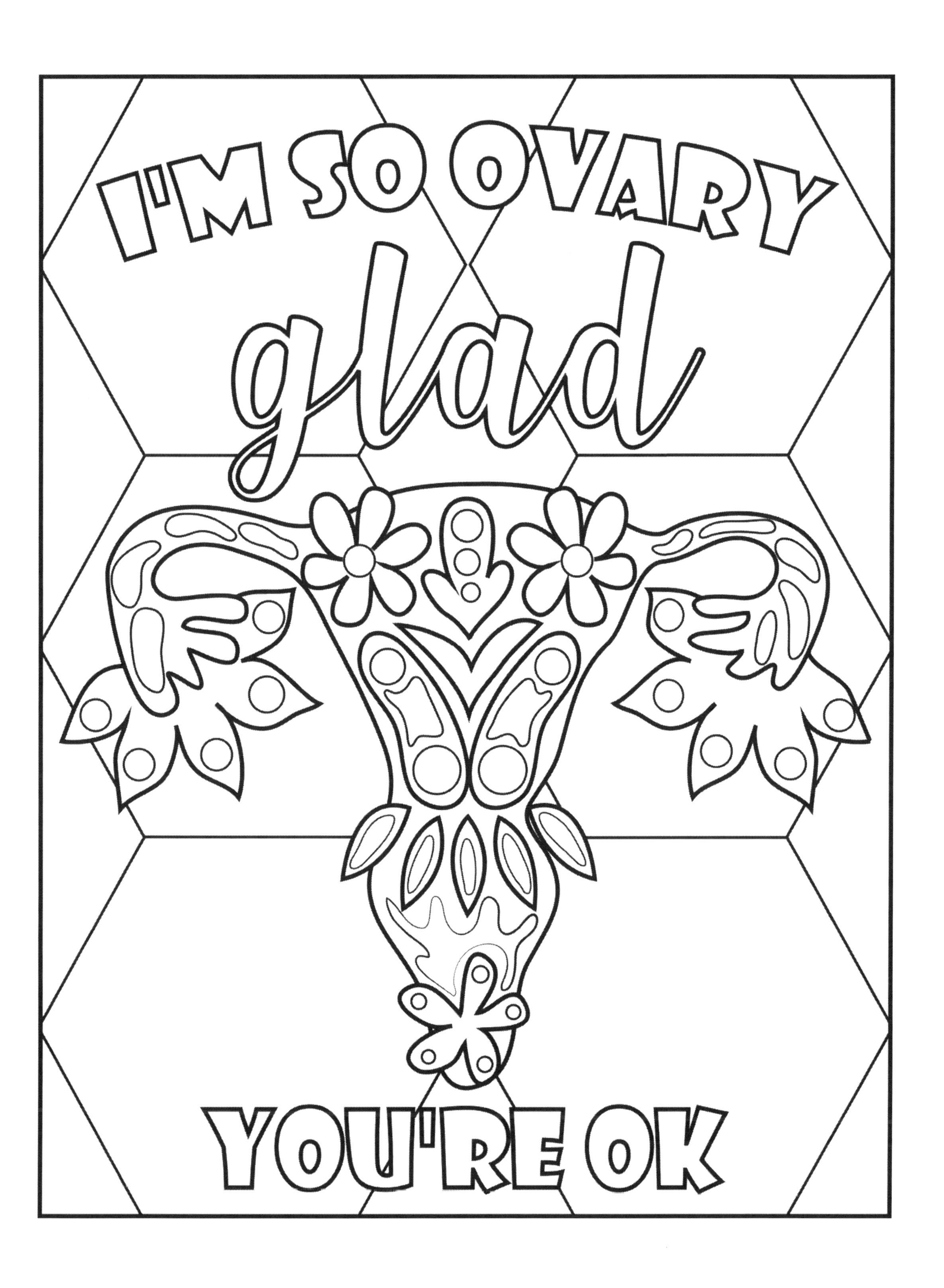
I'M SO OVARY
glad
YOU'RE OK

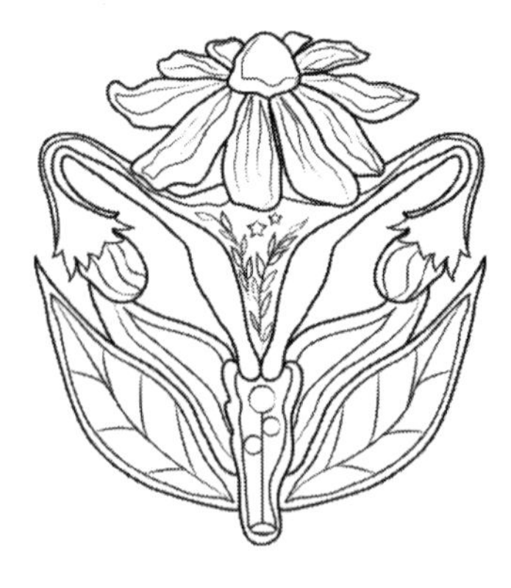

Buffer paper

Please cut and use between pages when you color with any ink that may cause bleeding.

This Page is Intentionally Left Blank.

Buffer paper

Please cut and use between pages when you color with any ink that may cause bleeding.

This Page is Intentionally Left Blank.

Made in United States
Troutdale, OR
01/19/2024

17026239R00042